1

"Fit, Healthy and Lean For Life"
(no gym required)

By:

Vsevolod (Seva) Berkolayko

"There are many open doors around us, you just need to open your eyes to see them."

Vsevolod (Seva) Berkolayko

Introduction

If you came across this book and you're presently reading this introduction, there's a good chance that you are ready to make some necessary changes in your life. Or, at the least, you're curious enough to see if changes can be made.

In any case, you're already working on the first step. By going out and seeking information, you become that much closer to your goal. I'll be blunt with this introduction, this book is plain and simple. You won't see any before or after pictures where people have lost tremendous weight and look completely different. There are no magic pills here either. As a matter a fact, I'm not highly supportive of supplements or any additional dietary supplements. In fact, you don't need any at all.

As a professional fighter who spent over ten years in the ring, I know a little something about getting into shape and obtaining a superior level of fitness. I have learned how to train my body and provide it with the proper nutrients needed to meet the physical goals that I've set for myself.

In this book I will equip you with the right tools and knowledge that you'll need to meet and exceed your fitness goals. Just looking good is not enough. You must feel one-hundred percent on the inside and out; therefore, that will indicate that you are completely healthy. Remember, you only get one body for a lifetime. Treat it well. Another helpful hint, if you mess up the one body you have, you'll end up regretting it for the rest of your life. Your body is not like a car, you can't replace it after a certain number of miles. The neglect or abuse will accumulate.

Whatever you do in this life, never just drag yourself through each day as if your very existence is inferior. No one has to have a monster ego, just be humble and be aware. Your awareness of your body will come with knowledge and experience.

Sedentary people pass away early and never achieve fulfillment in their lives. With this book, I want to show you how to take control of your life to prolong it and enjoy it. What would it be like to feel energetic, constantly happy and confident about your existence. Kind of interesting, huh? Well, everything written in this book, I actually apply to my own life. So we're not talking about the next guru fad, or the latest craze in fitness. The contents of this book are sincerely applicable to your life right now. I will only relate information that I have personally experienced myself and that I know works.

Secrets to Health & Longevity

What is health?

Health is a state of the organism where all of its functions are carried out quickly and effectively. It's a state of comfort, lightness, an ability to receive food, move around and execute all of life's functions.

It's a state that is reached owing to the working harmony of your bodies organs. It's a state when all the organs freely execute their functions pain free. If the stomach and the intestines effectively carry out the task of digestion and assimilation of food, if the heart and circulatory system are in good shape and provide good blood circulation, if the lungs provide the necessary inflow of oxygen to the blood, if the brain provides all its important functions, and the skin perspires easily, those are the main indications of health. In that case, we don't experience an unwell disposition or feelings of pain. We can carry out all the expected activities that are required. To be in that state is a supreme blessing and joy. Mother nature graciously allows us to preserve all of our organs and body parts in their original healthy state. If of course, we look after them and not do them undue harm, and therefore stay healthy. But if we don't bother to preserve the health of the organs, we won't be able to stay healthy.

Health is an equilibrium of the three elements in the body: breathing, bile and mucus under the conditions that the brain and bodily organs are working in harmony and order. The person is calm and happy, carrying out all of the responsibilities easily and freely. It's a state when a person sleeps good, has a good appetite and digestion, has a normal pulse, steady breathing, and a good amount of clean blood, nerves of steel, peaceful soul, and sparkling eyes. It's that state when a person wants to sing, jump, smile, laugh and move around with ease and joy. It's that state where we can think, speak and follow directions.

Good health is indeed a supreme blessing. What is the point of wealth and materialistic gain if a person can't eat well due to a sick stomach, if they can't walk because of rheumatism or palsy, or if they can't enjoy the beauty of nature because of a cataract or other eye illnesses? Life without good health is miserable and crippled , even for those who rule the world.

Good health, that's happiness, good health is wealth and it's life's potion. Without health, there's no joy. Without it, you cannot make a good living, you can't reach your desired goals, you simply can't give your best. Without health, there's no enthusiasm to work, and life becomes a burden. That's why preserving your health and the attention that goes with it, is paramount.

Without good health you won't be able to reach anything in the materialistic or spiritual world. Good health is an object of the most powerful desire, to maintain it occurs by or through living a natural lifestyle.

Health is not just an absence of illness, healthy people can fulfill a bigger volume of physical and mental labor/tasks as opposed to the unhealthy one. They can be deep in thought and meditation. Yet, healthy people are not necessarily physically strong or muscular and being physically strong or muscular does not mean that you are healthy. Health is a gift from Mother Nature or God, meaning that the power which nourishes all living beings. With birth we receive health, not illness. To be healthy is just as natural for a person as it is to live in general.

Good health is more valuable than gold and countless riches. It expands your soul, making it more receptive, therefore making you more cognizant of the essence of things. The one who has good health has no regrets. Actually, they generally tend to be truly happy people.

Health is the base of your career, but in reality the base of your whole life. To be completely healthy is when your body, mind and soul are working with each other in harmony. That's when you can enjoy life to the fullest capacity. When you easily handle your daily tasks and overcome obstacles. Without good health you won't be able to reach any of those things. Without it, you won't be able to fulfil selfless deeds. In old scriptures it is said ... "that our body is a boat, which we use to cross the ocean of earthly existence."

Science of Relaxation

Life in our days has become extremely difficult. In all aspects of life, there is unhealthy competition and a race for survival. People are going through many obstacles on a daily basis. Therefore, because of unhealthy life styles and poor ways of development, the human population is facing a lot of physical and mental stress.

People have developed a lot of unnatural habits, and forget the habits that were given to them by nature. Most muscles and nerves of a person are overlooked due to incorrect posture. Now they have to reacquire the knowledge from animals or even infants.

If you will practice relaxation, you will eliminate the loss of energy and will be active and energetic. During relaxation, muscles and nerves are resting. The energy accumulates in your body. Most who are not familiar with this wonderful science of relaxation are simply wasting away their energy, and subjecting their muscles and nerves to excessive loads, because they are doing unnecessary movements. Some people pointlessly rock their legs when sitting in a chair, some drum their fingers on a desk, some whistle, and some shake their heads. Because of not knowing the elementary principles of relaxation. The energy scatters due to the unnecessary movement of different body parts.

Fatigue is a result of excessively overloading different body parts. If you are going through intense studying or an intellectual task, it could be the brain or, it could be the body if you are running around doing various tasks the entire day. On top of that, you may burn down the neural energy as well. If something happens which causes a burst of emotions, you can experience a rough reaction, and soon afterwards you feel tired. That's why you have to learn to relax and take breaks during the day, rather than just at night.

The first sign that your brain is tired is when no matter how hard you try, you're unable to focus your attention on whatever you are doing. The brain needs rest and relaxation, in order for you to be able to concentrate on your work, or a specific task. In order to stay healthy, it's necessary to do physical exercises. But relaxation is just as important.

Complete relaxation is what you reach during sleep. When your sleep is disturbed, or you experience nightmares, these interruptions prevent your body from having the chance to gain complete relaxation. Actually, even after a long night sleep, a person generally still wakes up tired.

You can maintain good health by alternating between sleep and relaxation. Only then, does the body tissue correctly consume blood, taking in nutrients, grow, rejuvenate and eliminate waste. Remember that laziness and idleness have nothing in common with relaxation. Lazy people are passive, they don't like to work. They struggle with sleep as opposed to the person who practices relaxation: who is energetic, strong, robust and vivacious. These people will never let even a little particle of energy go to waste. That person can work for long periods, quickly and effectively.

When you feel sleepy, that means that your organs need to rest. Give that rest to your body and brain at the same time. A few minutes of relaxation will remarkably refresh you and restore energy. And once again, you can effectively carry on with your tasks. Learn to fall asleep when you need to at any time. You can practice relaxation when you are awake and even when you are working. Not all body parts work at the same time. While certain tissues are working, you can give rest to others. You should really learn the science of relaxation. The quality of relaxation depends on the mentality or the persons temper. The one who gets disturbed easily won't be able to relax correctly. His/her sleep is always restless and full of bad dreams.

Relaxation comes as a result of discipline. Busy people like lawyers and doctors must know the science of relaxation. They should practice this concept every day in order to always be alert in the place of business. You can relax your body and mind at the train station or sitting on a bench in a park. Relaxing completely refreshes the person.

Yogis learned this science to the fullest. They practice it to perfection. Those who have command of this art can preserve and accumulate their mental and physical energy, and to use it effectively later on. Even standing up, they can close their eyes for a few minutes and regain enough energy to keep on going. When they are in a relaxed phase, the energy flows through their nerves like water flows through a pipe. Those who don't know how to relax are vainly wasting their mental and physical energy.

When you want your muscles to contract in order to execute some type of activity, impulse from the brain is transmitted through the nerves to the muscles. Energy goes through the nerves, reaching the muscles and causes them to contract. When the muscles contracts, it brings to movement that certain part of the body which you choose to activate. For example: when you want to lift a chair, that command is created by an impulse in the brain. The brain transmits this through the nerves to the arms muscles. Direct energy currents travel through the nerves from the brain. Muscles contract and execute the necessary action in order to lift the chair. All other activities such as the conscious and unconscious are executed in the same fashion. If the muscles are overworked, more energy is consumed, and you feel more fatigued. Muscles wear out because of an overload, or over exertion due to loss of great amounts of energy.

Unconscious actions are carried out on instinct. Your consciousness does not wait for orders. If a dog bites you on the hand, you will instantly jerk your hand away. There is no doubt or hesitation at that time. This is your instinct, which is a mechanical reaction.

An action of your muscle groups may be controlled with the aid of others. One impulse may activate one muscle group, but if you send another suppressing impulse through a different muscle group, you counteract the first one. For example: if someone picks on you and insults you, you can jump up in order to beat them up. In other words, an impulse is already activating a specific muscle group. But you can control that impulse by analyzing and thinking "I won't gain anything by hurting this idiot, it's simply not worth it," I'd rather forgive them and let it go. The counteracting impulse will instantly stop the first muscle group. Impulses, counter impulses or constraint impulses cause the nerves, muscles and brain to work intensively. Most people are the slaves of their own impulses, and therefore are lacking spiritual peace.

A woman who cannot relax and properly rest will not preserve her beauty. Body fatigue symptoms will occur on her face. The body itself is going to lose the perfection of shape. Constant stress, which is common amongst women, can age her quickly, diminish her natural beauty, and force her to realize that her strength has decreased. Science of Relaxation is an exact science and simple to learn muscle relaxation is as important as it's contracting. I pay specific attention to relaxation of the mind, where nerves as well as muscles can relax together.

There are two types of relaxation: mental and physical. There's also another classification. If you relax only some muscles in certain body parts, that's partial relaxation. If you relax the muscles of the whole body, that's total relaxation. If you will be able to completely relax all the muscles, nerves and brain, you will automatically fall into deep sleep. Some people who master this technique can fall asleep at any time. They can do this day or night, as well as when they wake up and when they choose to. This can really come in handy at work, when you can fall asleep in a chair, at your desk or in a few minutes, even if your surrounded by a lot of noise.Those who have a perfect balance within their mind are able to relax and fall asleep at any time.

A few minutes of relaxation will help you regain your strength. Once in the morning and then again after dinner, you should practice relaxation for about ten minutes at a minimum. Regardless of whether you're busy or in a rush, you need to follow this habit religiously. Sit in a comfortable chair or lay down, put a pillow under your knees. The legs should be about eighteen inches away from the floor and allow all your muscles to "deflate", sort of speak. If you are laying down, put a pillow under your head, it will help your neck relax. Close your eyes. Create a vacuum in your consciousness.

The legs have to be slightly lifted in order for the spine to be straight while also allowing blood to flow away from the legs. If you are sitting in a chair, place your legs on an elevated surface and relax all muscles; it won't be easy at first, but with time, it will turn into a habit.

Never sit on the edge of the chair, lean back and place a hard pillow behind your lower back. Don't cross your legs. With your feet pressed firmly against the surface, keep the knees and feet together. Exhaustion can also be avoided by getting into a correct posture when you stand. If you have to stand on your feet most of the time, due to your job for example, then bring your knees and ankles together when you stand. That way you can create a single post on which your body rests. That way the weight of the body does not transfer on one leg, but equally distributes onto both legs.

Mental Relaxation

Just like you relax your muscles after the exercise, you also have to relax your mind and give it a rest. Muscle relaxation gives rest to the mind. Relaxation of the mind gives rest to the body. The body is a shape that the mind casts for its own pleasure.

The mind accumulates experiences with the aid of the body and works together with the energy senses of the body. The mind influences the body. For example: if you are happy, your body feels strong and healthy as well, when you are depressed, your body can't function properly. The body has a certain influence on the mind as well. If the body is healthy and strong, you're feeling happy and energetic. If you are in pain, the mind can't function properly either. Thoughts take shape of effect, the effect influences the mind. If you take away the tension from your muscles, you bring ease and peacefulness to the mind.

An easily agitated person can't have mental peace. The brain, nerves and muscles are always under constant stress every minute a person wastes muscle, nerve and brain energy. People like this are weak, even if they possess a lot of physical strength, and simply because he/she easily loses the mental balance. If you really want to enjoy peace and constant joy, eliminate the worries, anxiety, fear and anger from your mind and control your impulses.

Worrying and getting mad for no reason won't give you any type of benefit. Fear, anger and anxiety are the products of ignorance. When you become a victim of anger, your muscles and nerves are always tensed. The nature of anger is rough and brutal. Anger causes unquestionable damage to the brain, blood and nerves. You have nothing positive to gain by displaying anger. Methods of the repetition of any type of action in the mind develops a habit. If you are often under stress you develop a habit of worrying. Your life energy is sucked out of you from anger, fear and stress. Why be afraid of anything, when there are so many good things in life you can enjoy?

Balance and peace within the mind can be reached by eliminating worries, fear and anger. Be aware and reasonable. Stay away from unnecessary worries. Excluding all the worries, fear and anger from your life. Concentrate on boldness, happiness, joy and peace of mind, great strength and vivacity.

Also remember, when you relax mentally or physically, your mind should not be occupied by any outside or incidental thoughts. Practicing mental relaxation will take away inner tension, and it will fill up your mind with new energy and will make you happy and cheerful.

Sleep

In order to be in good health, you must get enough rest. In nature everything is cyclical. A period of activity always shifts to a period of inaction. Even the heart has intervals when it rests between the beats. Sleep is the most absolute way of rest. This is when all the tissues are completely resting. Muscles are totally relaxed. The heart contractions slow down and the brain is resting as well. Just like night replaces the day, in return, work must be replaced with rest.

During a rest period, the tissues are being renewed and rejuvenated. The best form of relaxation is reached through sleep. Then nature takes a person into its bosom to wash off the fatigue of the brain and nerves. To rejuvenate and give yourself energy and a good spirit, you may continue with your activities the next day if you have restful sleep. Sleep is a physiological occurrence where your mind, brain and organs get a few hours of rest. It's a natural toner necessary for a healthy life style. The more soundly you sleep, the healthier you're going to be. The number of necessary hours of sleep depends on your physical and mental needs. This allows you not to struggle with fatigue. Without the sufficient amount of sleep, you won't be able to function properly. The older the person gets the less sleep they require. Most people over sixty years of age get enough sleep within six hours, as opposed to children who need to sleep nine to ten hours daily.

As for the rest of us, seven to eight hours is just about right. Sleeping too much is a very unhealthy habit as well. It causes a person to be sluggish and inactive. The most important aspect about sleep is the quality of sleep you get. Even if you go into a deep sound sleep without any dreams for only a few hours, you will wake up completely refreshed. There isn't any type of benefit if you roll around your bed for hours, you will only get irritated and won't get any quality rest.

Sleeping too long is not good for you either. It causes early aging and weakens your mental abilities. This is the same as going to bed too late in the evening. Also, you should avoid sleeping during the day, especially after a meal. This can cause dyspepsia or indigestion as well as kidney illness.

It's better to sleep with an open window, the more clean air you inhale during sleep the more cheerful you will feel when you wake up the next day. Try not to take any sleeping pills. If you have a problem falling asleep, go take a walk outside for fifteen minutes and then go to bed right afterward. Chances are you will fall asleep shortly. Sleep on your side, preferably on the left, this helps digestion. Try going to sleep at the same time every night, wear loose garments. Don't cover yourself completely with heavy quilts, especially don't fall asleep with your head underneath the blankets. This is very unhygienic. You will inhale the spoiled oxygen, which already has passed through your lungs. Candles, lamps and fire places pollute the air, all of those must be turned off or put out before going to bed.

Do not eat before going to bed. Late dinner forces your brain to work and distorts your sleep. The brain is going to have to participate in the work of digestion instead of maintaining sleep at that time. If you want sound sleep, you must keep a regimen of your food intake. For example: if you're going to bed at nine p.m., your last meal should be at six o'clock. Don't build castles in the sky when trying to fall asleep. Don't create any plans or schedules for the next day. If you're mad at someone, just let it go. Think of good thoughts. Let them sink deep into your consciousness, and you will have a good night's sleep without any disturbing dreams. When you begin falling asleep, first your eyelids begin to close. The brain does not receive any visual signals or impressions. The sense of smell and taste leave you and later on, the sense of hearing as well. At last, your whole being falls into sleep.

Sleep, as a state of relaxation should not be turned into a strict frame of regulations. After all, a lot depends on the individuals physical and mental strengths. It also depends on your body's constitution, volume of executed tasks as well as the type of activities you're engaged in throughout the day. For example: people that engage in mental labor need more rest and sleep than those who are occupied with mainly physical work. Those who are of age should decide for themselves how much sleep they may need.

Exercise

Why Exercise?

Physical exercise is essential in all phases of life, especially during childhood and adolescent years. Exercise is very important in maintaining good health, strength and energy, as well as supports a healthy balance for the organs. Exercise increases the working effectiveness of the body and mind. It improves your ability and desire to communicate and collaborate with others. It also helps you control your weaknesses and allows freedom for your soul. Exercise keeps unnecessary weight off and improves the weak aspects of one's body. It can also help your body rehabilitate faster after illness.

Exercise is very important for all the organs contained within the body, in order for them to function effectively. It's necessary to maintain growth and tissue replacement and provide enough oxygen to the entire body. Without physical exercise, you cannot have good health. Your entire system will not function properly. The stomach won't digest food efficiently and your blood will be full of toxic substances and free radicals. The heart cannot function effectively without certain types of exercise. If you train the heart constantly, it will pump blood more intensely, and the lungs will inhale more frequently. More air will be exhaled and unnecessary compounds eliminated from the body and the thorax will also get wider. If the heart function gets better as a result of exercise, the blood stagnation disappears as well as the risk of congested vessels. The blood will be distributed evenly and improve the circulatory system and the lungs functions. The amount of waste expelled out of the lungs will be greatly increased. Exercise gives your whole body a healthy appearance. It provides a fast blood current, stimulates the kidneys, lungs, and skin, which withdraws harmful substances. It also helps to carry out a cleansing of your body quickly and effectively. Muscular exercise has a positive effect on your whole body. It helps to get rid of constipation and normalizes the bowels movements. It improves the mind and the quality of mental labor. It improves skin functions, which result from an increase in perspiration that cause the body to regulate and decreases your body' s temperature.

All body movements are produced with the help of the muscles. That which gives them growth and energy. If you have well developed muscles, you can execute more tasks easier and more effectively. If you do not exercise, chances are your muscles are weak and underdeveloped. You won't have any endurance. If one of the body's organs is not being used, little by little they become less efficient and will atrophy. For example, if you brake your leg and wear a cast for a month, when the cast comes off, the recently broken leg is going to be smaller than a healthy one. This occurs because the muscles haven't been used during this time, but if the muscles are constantly working, they will increase in size. Look at most professional athletes, they all have well developed looking physiques. Although, strength and size cannot be equated every time.   However, a muscular person and a thin person can be equally strong.

You must have nicely developed muscles without the outward sign of excess fat. Overweight people are forced to carry extra loads on their entire skeletal frame. It takes more energy for them and they will tend to get tired more because of the excess weight and stored wastes within their bodies. To burn fat, you need to do regular and systematic exercises. The exercises should be chosen and adapted towards the needs and abilities of your body. Don't jump into overly intensive workouts right away. Take it slow, allow your body to adapt to the physical exertion. While exercising, don't get to the point where you are overly fatigued. In that case, it usually means you are doing more than your body can handle. Extremely hard exercise might not be good at first either. This will do more harm than good, potentially causing injuries. Add more exercises when you feel that your regular workout is too easy for you. Only you will know how far you can push yourself. Learn to listen to your body and don't be lazy. Your ideal body is in your own hands.

Stretching

Stretching before a workout is very important for several reasons. When you stretch, you warm the muscles up properly and increase the range of motion to obtain maximum blood flow, which will allow you to completely benefit from the workout ahead. A warm and stretched muscle can execute exercise much easier than muscles that are cold and unresponsive. Working out without proper stretching can cause pain and injuries. Inflexible tendons and other tissues tend to shrink, this increases the chances of pulling a muscle or causing an injury. This insufficient approach may put you out of commission for several days or even weeks if not properly evaluated.

On the other hand, regular stretching helps you stay flexible for future use. Usually after thirty, people lose one percent of their flexibility every year, so by the time you reach sixty, you're going to be thirty percent less flexible. Regular stretching will greatly slow down this inevitable process. Flexibility is one of the key ingredients to staying young. Ten to fifteen minutes a day is more than enough for a full body stretch session. Hold each specific stretch for fifteen to twenty seconds and take deep breaths to help you relax and expel tension throughout your body. This will help you avoid discomfort. Make this an everyday routine, and you will see great improvements in your everyday life activities.

Head Roll

Keep your feet at shoulder width with your arms at your sides. Slowly lower your head forward, then roll it to the left, backward and to the right in a circular motion. Do this five times, then go through this in the opposite direction.

Shoulder Roll

Keep your feet at shoulder width with arms at your sides. Shrug your shoulders up and roll them forward and down, then back and up in a circular motion five times on each side.

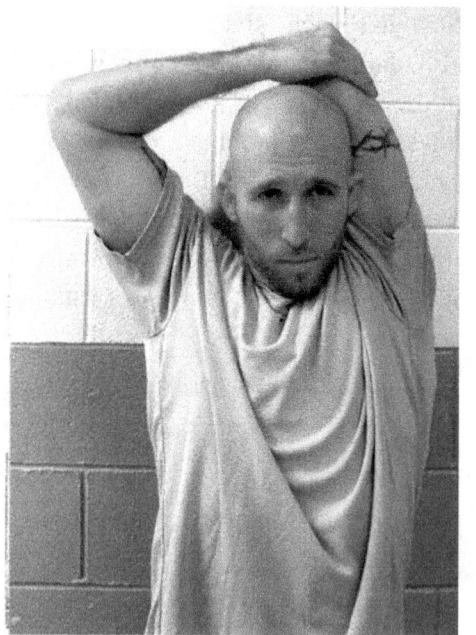

Horizontal Elbow Stretch

Keep your feet at shoulder width with one leg forward. Extend your left arm forward and bend at the elbow so the tip of your fingers touch the back of your neck. Put your right hand on the back of the left elbow and press as far as your left arm can go. Hold for ten seconds, switch arms.

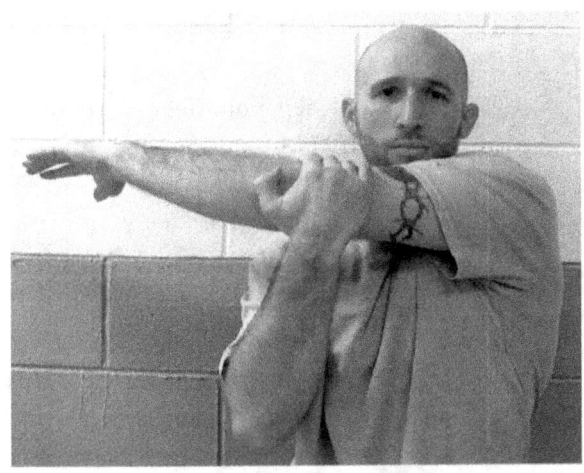

Vertical Elbow Stretch

Keep your feet at shoulder width with one leg forward. Raise your left arm and bend at the elbow. Put your right hand on the back of the left elbow and press as far as your left arm can go. Hold for ten seconds, switch arms.

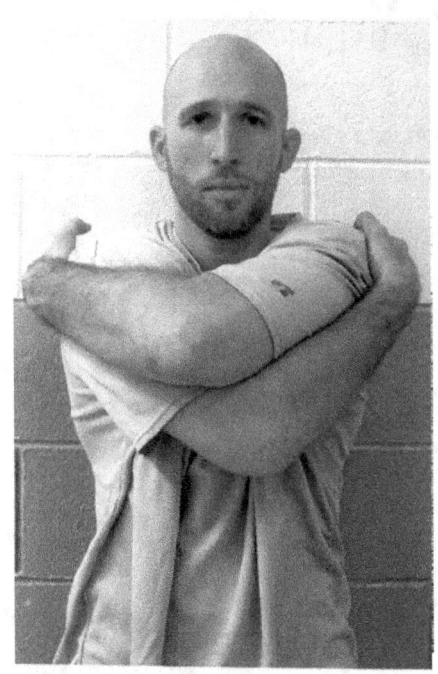

Hugger Stretch

Keep your feet at shoulder width with your arms extended out to your sides and parallel to the floor. Quickly throw your arms around your torso in a hugging motion, then quickly open and extend your arms as wide as possible.

Then throw your arms around your torso once again, switching the arm positions from top to bottom. Repeat, fifteen to twenty times.

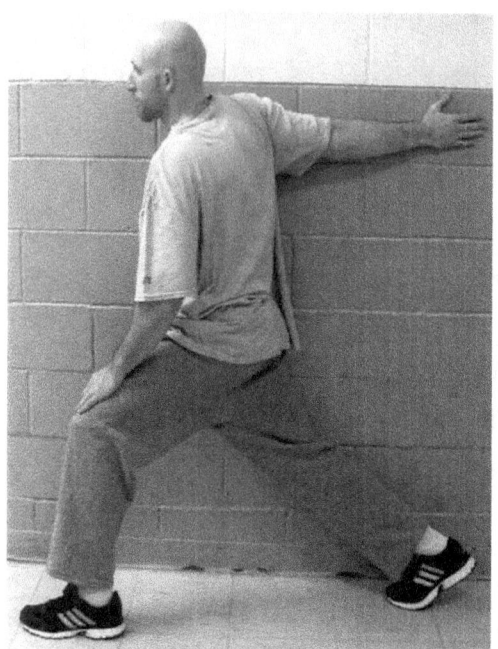

Wall Stretch-

Keep your feet at shoulder width with one leg forward. Face a wall and extend an arm against it. Your palm should be open and flat against the wall.

Keep your arm in this position and slowly turn your upper body away from the wall as far as you can.

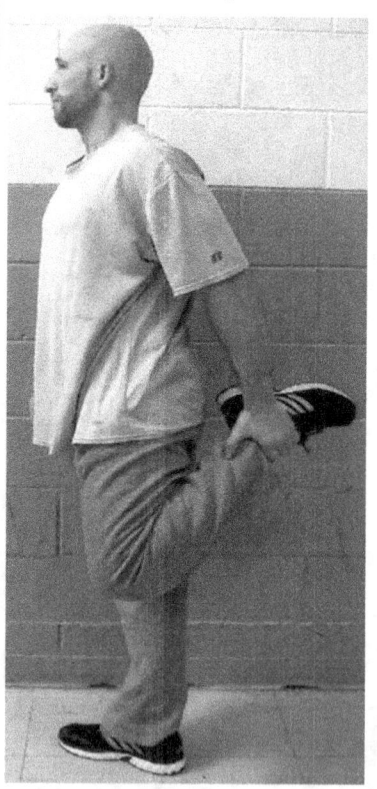

Hold this position for twenty seconds, then switch arms.

Quad Stretch -

Stand on one foot and bend the other knee. While using the same side hand, grab the top of your foot and pull it up toward your butt.

Hold this position for fifteen seconds, then switch legs.

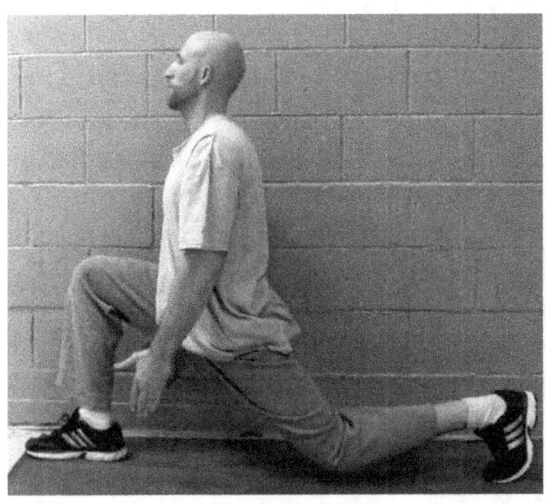

Runner's Stretch -

Get into a lunge position with your left knee bent and your right leg straight and sturdy as you drive the back heel toward the floor. Lift your chest away from your thigh. Move your hands so that your fingertips are barely touching the floor, with your arms straight. Look forward and hold this position for fifteen seconds then repeat on the opposite side.

Lunge Stretch -

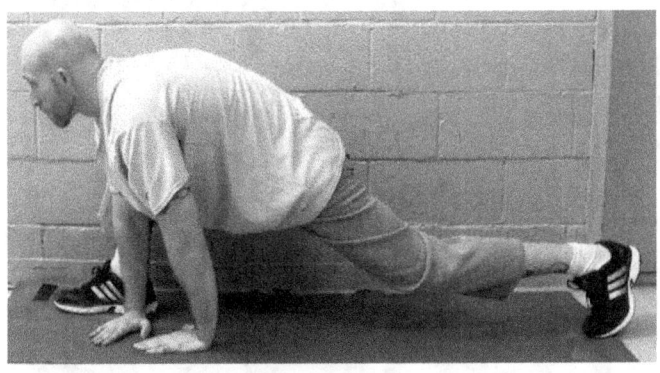

Get into a lunge position with your left knee bent and your right leg straight. Put your hands on the floor on the inside of your left foot. Drop your pelvis as low as possible while keeping your back leg straight. Hold this position for fifteen seconds and then change legs.

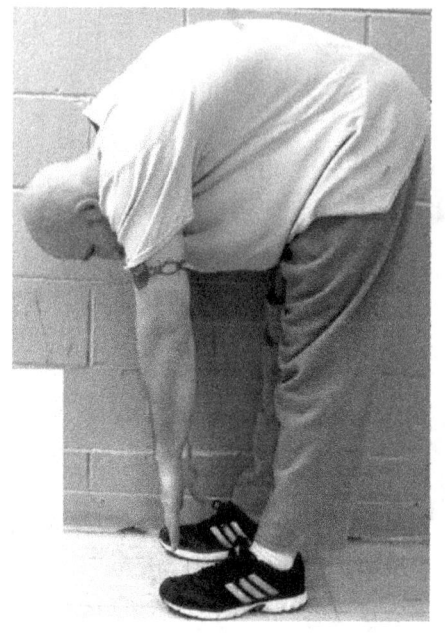

Hamstring Stretch -

Stand straight, your feet hip-width and arms at your sides with feet parallel. Take a deep breath with your arms straight over head. Exhale, folding forward at the hips and touch your toes. Go as far as possible and hold this position for twenty seconds.

If you cannot touch your toes, extend as far as possible.

Side Stretch -

Stand with your feet slightly more than shoulder width apart. Bend to the left reaching your right hand over your head, stretching the right side of your body, while keeping your left hand on your thigh.

Hold this position for fifteen seconds, then repeat this movement to your right, stretching your left side.

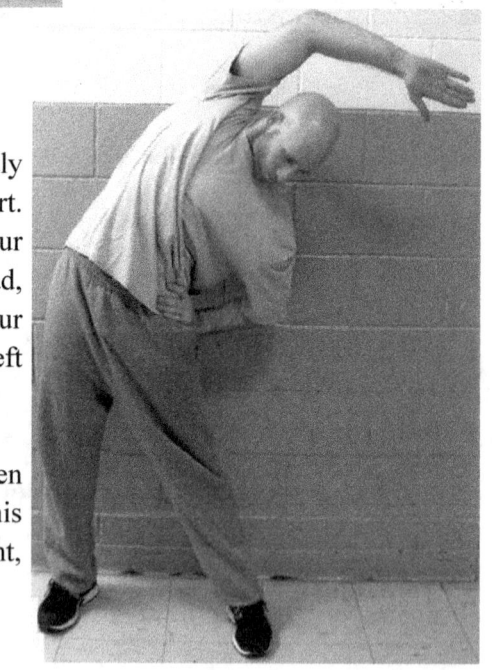

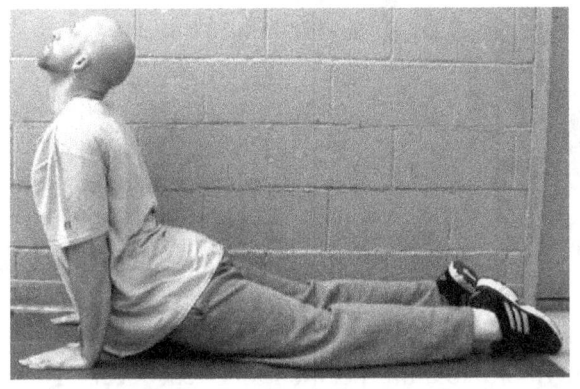

Cobra Stretch -

Lower yourself to the bottom of a push-up position.

Keep your hands shoulder width apart and arms straight, perpendicular to the floor. With your wrists directly beneath your shoulders, slowly lift your head and upper body.

Try your best to keep your lower body touching the floor. Relax your back and look up. - Hold this position for ten seconds.

Infants Stretch -

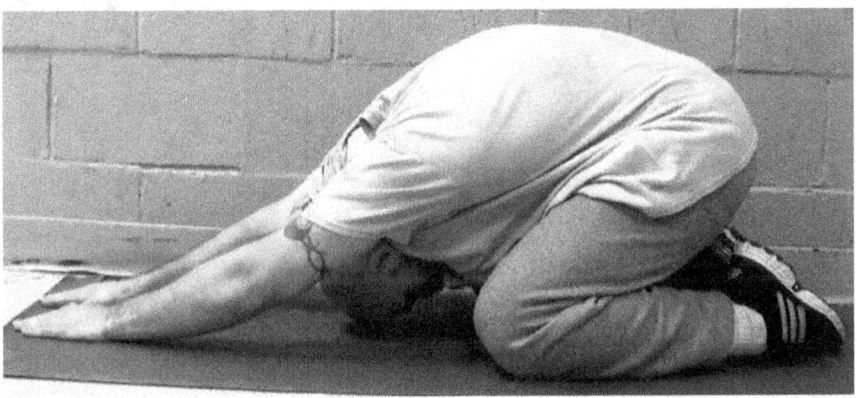

Kneel on the floor with your knees slightly wider than hip-width apart and your big toes touching behind you. Bring your forehead down onto the floor. Reach forward with both arms placing the palms flat on the floor. Relax your body and hold this position for twenty seconds.

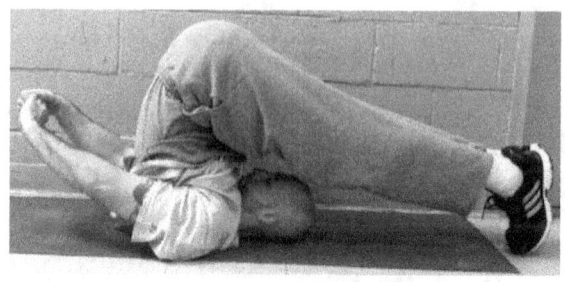

The Plough Stretch

Lay down straight on your back. Keep your palms touching your sides with both legs together and slowly bring them up with your knees straight. Try to keep your arms on the floor and body straight. Then slowly lower both legs behind your head until your toes touch the floor. Hold this position for twenty seconds.

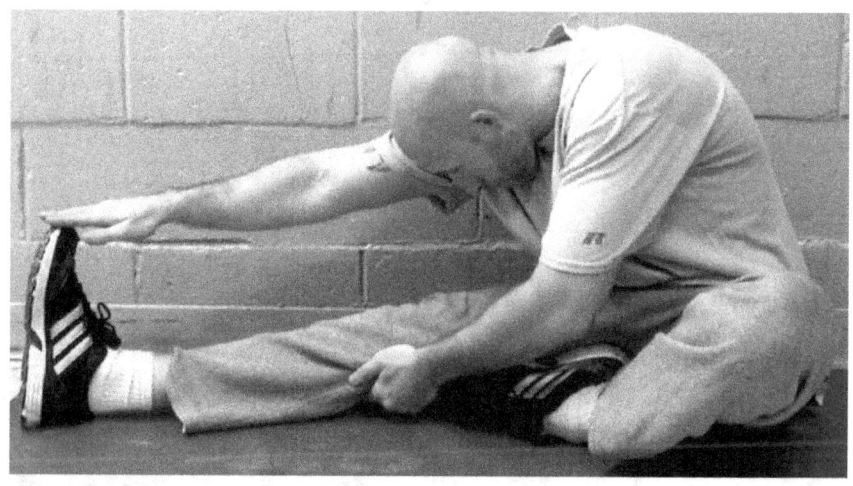

Head to Knee Stretch

Sit on the floor. Straighten out your right leg and bend your left knee, so the bottom of your left foot touches the inner thigh of your right leg. Slowly bend towards your right foot as far as you can go and try to place your forehead onto your right knee.

Hold this position for ten to fifteen seconds, then repeat on the opposite side.

Butterfly Stretch-

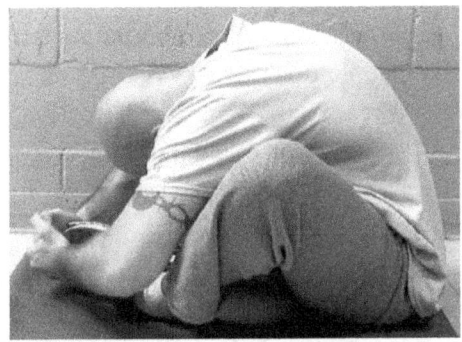

Sit up straight in a seated position with the bottom of your feet together and your knees out to the sides. Place your feet about five inches away from your body. Lean forward and try to touch your feet with your forehead, while keeping your hands on top of your feet in the same position.

Hold this position for twenty to thirty seconds.

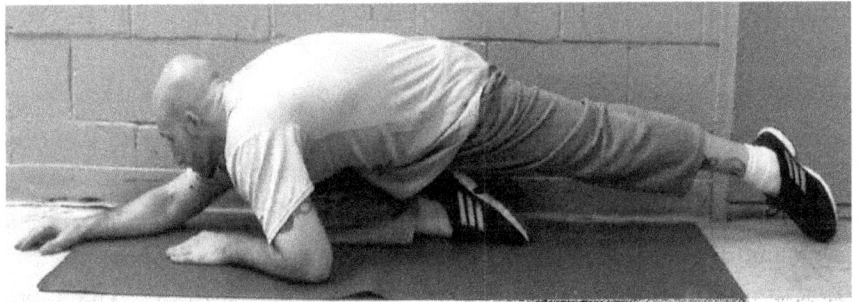

T-Stretch

Get on your knees, pull the right knee to the outside of your right hand with your foot under the groin as your shin and ankle touch the floor. Extend your left leg straight behind you, allowing the top of your foot to touch the floor. Bring your forehead close to the floor with your right arm reaching out in front of you.

Hold this position for thirty seconds then repeat on the opposite side.

Cardio

When you think of doing cardiovascular or cardio-pulmonary activity, what comes to mind? Most people don't really have any idea. Forget what you think you know and realize that your cardio activity should be the basis for all of your other activities. Mental or physical, it doesn't matter, cardio activity deliver's fresh, oxygenated blood to the entire body.

This improves the body's total ability to function at peak efficiency. Cardio activity cleanses the blood of toxins and free radicals. So ask yourself this question, will my body and mind perform better if my blood flows more efficiently (better blood pressure as well) and my lungs can process and distribute oxygen more effectively?

If you lead an active lifestyle and would like to improve your capabilities or maintain better health, you should incorporate a cardio regimen into your training. Whether you're a weight lifter, boxer, professional athlete or just a novice exercise enthusiast, cardio training can improve your overall health and personal goals, as well as burn body fat for that lean physique everyone is trying to achieve. The more intense your cardio is the more body fat you'll ultimately burn. Over time you'll burn more body fat from more intense cardio than you will from longer sessions of leisurely/steady pace cardio. Intense cardio revs up your body's metabolic rate much higher for longer periods of time then steady state cardio. And, you'll burn much more body fat in the hours after you finish intense cardio, rather during the same time frame doing leisurely cardio for a longer duration. But personally, I believe twenty to thirty minutes of cardio is just right, unless you're a professional athlete or require a greater amount. Also, for greater fat loss strategies, cut the carbohydrates before your cardio routine. When you take in carbs, particularly in the form of sugar, they go directly into your bloodstream, making them immediately available for use as energy. And your body will tend to burn off these calories first before it taps into your fat stores. To get to those fat stores much sooner, the key is to avoid taking in carbs for up to two hours before you perform cardio sessions, a technique that allows your body to burn stored fat instead. One of the best times of the day to burn body fat through cardio is when you first wake up, because you have little glucose in your system. Remember, you haven't eaten since the night before so your body is literally running on empty. Because of this, you may need some calories to get through your workouts. If so, rely on protein with or without dietary fats. You can have a no carb protein shake or consume whole foods like eggs, chicken breast, fish or cottage cheese.

Even a table spoon of natural peanut-butter will do. So, which form of cardio is right for you? I would say swimming is great, but not everyone has an Olympic swimming pool in their backyard. So I can suggest jogging, whether its outside or on a treadmill. It's a great way to burn fat or even better, a stair climber. This is a simple exercise you can perform anywhere. There is a staircase wherever, at home or out in the public. You've likely seen films depicting athletes running up large staircases in stadiums before, and this is because it's great exercise. It's especially effective if you skip every other step. Not only is it great cardio but stair climbing is absolutely great exercise in general. This is a type of exercise that strengthens your leg muscles.

Basically , a cardio workout does not have to consist of running or aerobics, there are things you can do throughout your day that make for great cardio exercise, and most of them don't even feel like training which means you're more likely to do them often and for long durations. And all that of course, leads up to more calories burned and more fat lost. There are just a few suggestions for other ways to have fun and burn fat while getting a good cardio workout. Bicycling, basketball, hiking, ice skating, racquetball, rollerblading, tennis, rowing or playing soccer. But if you are a busy bee and really don't have much time to step out, here are some cardio exercises you can do in the comfort of your own home or even at work during a lunch break.

Jumping Jacks- stand with your feet together and hands at your sides. Clap your hands after you raise your arms above your head. Jump up just enough to be able to spread your feet wide. Without pausing, quickly reverse the movement and repeat.

Jumping Rope- This exercise develops fast twitch muscle fibers with one-fifth the impact of running. Just ten minutes burns almost double the calories of jogging and improves footwork for sports like soccer, basketball and martial arts. Stand tall and jump rope, landing on both feet, get to the point where you can string several successful reps together. The most intense rhythm is a single jump per revolution. A good alternative is a slight bounce between jumps, you can also place one foot in front of the other, rocking back and forth, just make sure to switch up your legs so that you work both sides equally. Another alternative is a "Boxer's jump rope", that's when you jump with one foot forward and one back, and switch your foot positions with each revolution. You'll still land on both feet simultaneously.

Burpee- perform this classic military/jail house drill for at least ten reps, striving to complete each rep with good form, (you can check out your positioning in a mirror, if you have one available). To perform a burpee: Start in a standing position then squat down and plant your hands on the floor. Shoot your legs behind you to find yourself in a push-up position. Perform a push-up, and then reverse the motion quickly to raise back up into the starting position. Jump up, stretching your hands over your head while holding your abdominals tight. Shadow boxing or some simple punch-kick combinations is also a great cardio workout. Not to mention you don't have to actually hit something to release tension, just putting power into attack motion, can actually help you return to your day much more relaxed after you're done training.

Burpee- 1

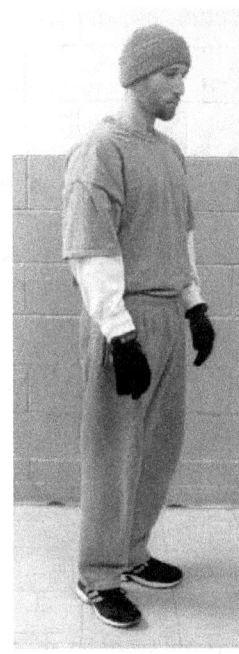

Burpee- 2

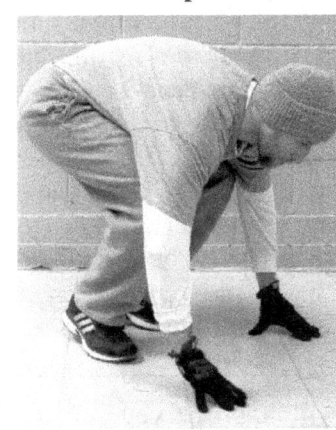

Burpee-3

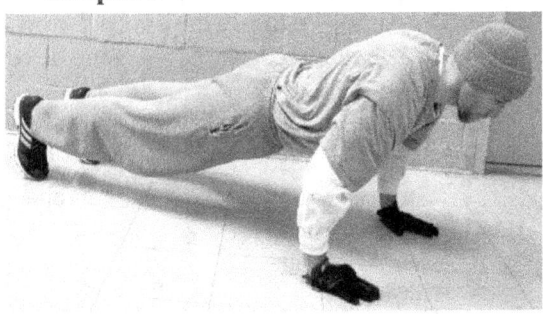

Burpee-4

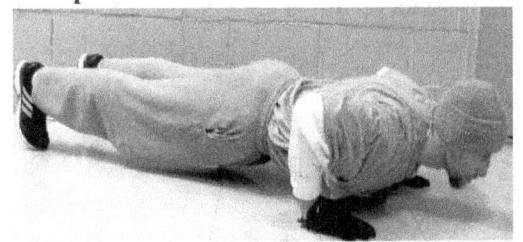

Burpee-5

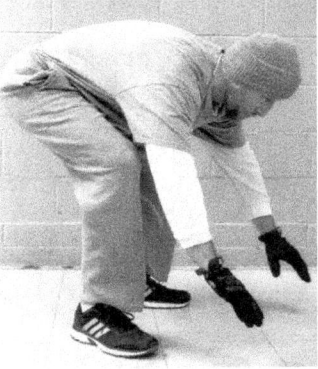

CORE

Your core is considered the epicenter of your entire body. Its importance in form and function cannot be overestimated. There are several reasons why it's important to have a strong core. For one thing, core applies to the muscle compartments of the abdominal area, side oblique muscles and lower back muscles as well. They all work together to stabilize and support the spine. The majority of backaches can be eliminated by strengthening your core muscles. Also, a strong core helps you gain strength and power in order to perform any kind of athletic exercises. When your core is strong, your whole body benefits. And finally, because the core encompasses all the abdominal muscles that make up that nice looking six pack, a strong core is the foundation for a ripped midsection.

In this chapter, I will offer you a variety of core exercises. Which will improve your posture and enhance movements used for daily activities as well as athletic performance. They will also help flatten your stomach and decrease excess back and belly fat. But if that doesn't make you a believer, here is ten general reasons why you should do core exercises.

1) Allows greater muscles stimulation through isometric holds.

2) Surpasses plateaus, as the body changes occur more quickly.

3) Increases the basal metabolic rate.

4) Improves mental focus and discipline.

5) Enhances muscle strength, stability and synergism.

6) Provides a great workout when postures are performed in rapid succession.

7) Burns more than six hundred calories in a typical ninety minute session.

8) Increases circulation and by extension, promotes vitality, immune function improvement and waste elimination.

9.) Creates enhanced and permanent physical changes.

10.) Promotes mental stability and serene feeling.

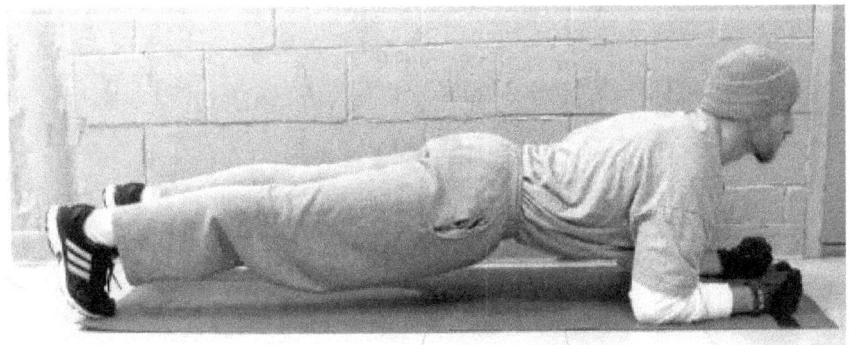

Plank Pose- Strengthens almost every muscle in your body from your shoulders to your calves, and your entire core-abs, lower back, and glutes. Lie down on your stomach, then prop yourself up on your elbows, bent at ninety degrees, shoulder width apart, allowing your forearms to relax on the ground. You may want to place your elbows on a yoga mat for comfort. Hold this position for as long as you can. It's good to start with one minute and gradually build it up to five.

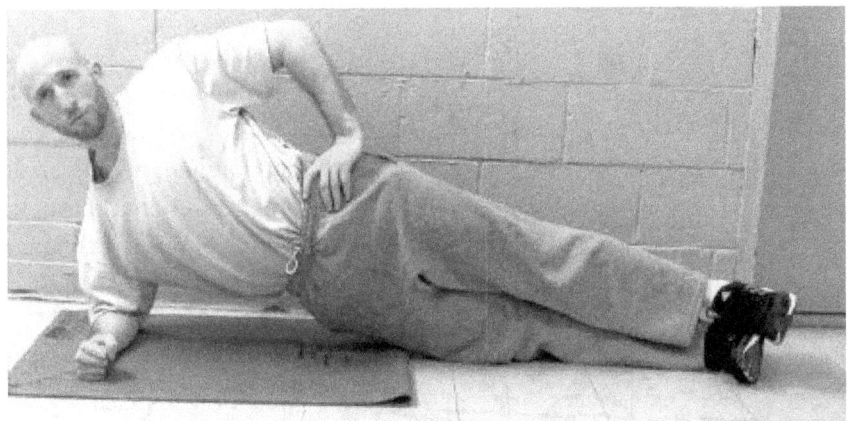

Side Plank-Tones every muscle from shoulders to ankles.

Lie on your right side with your right elbow directly underneath your shoulder. Place your left foot on top of your right foot. Now raise your pelvis off the ground so that your body's straight from head to heel and your pelvis is forward and in line with the rest of your body. Hold this position for one minute to two minutes, then switch sides.

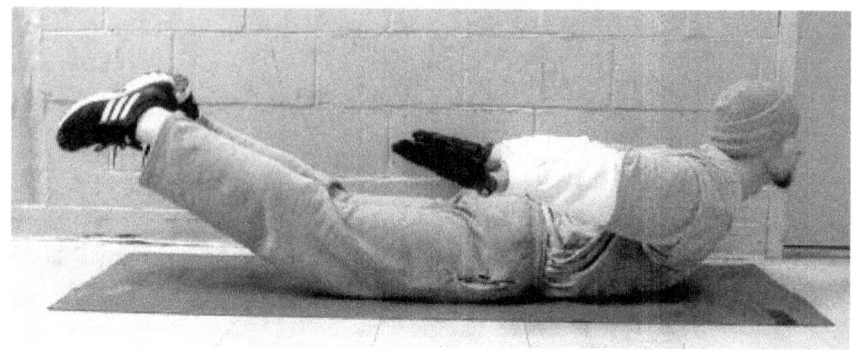

Locust Pose-Tones glutes, hamstrings and lower back.
Lie down flat on your stomach with your arms extended beside the body with the back of the hands on the floor. Keeping your legs and arms straight, lift them all off the ground as high as possible, so that only your torso and pelvis are still on the ground. Hold this pose for five seconds and repeat three times.

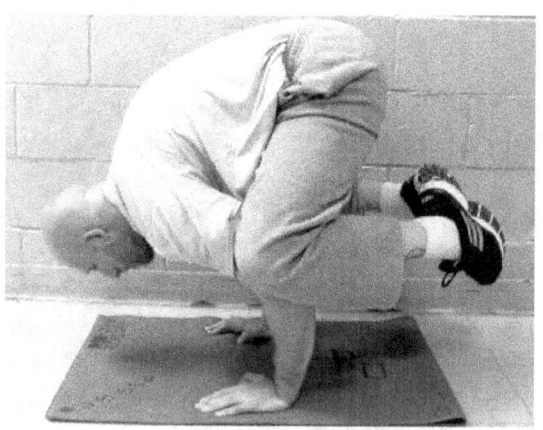

Crane Pose -
Strengthens the wrists, arms, shoulders, and abdominal muscles. It requires concentration and helps you conquer the fear of falling forward.

From a crouched position, place your hands shoulder width apart on the floor. Open your knees wider than your elbows and press the inside of your knees against your upper arms. Shift your weight onto your hands and slowly lift one foot at a time off the floor until you find your balance point. Hold this position for as long as you can maintain your balance.

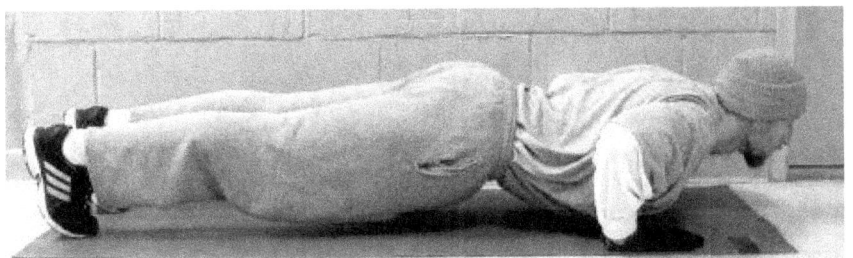

Crocodile Pose-Strengthens the arms, wrists, shoulders and tones the abdomen. Lie on the floor on your stomach. Bend the elbows, place the hands on the floor with fingers pointing forward and tuck the toes under yourself. Flex your abs and lift your whole body approximately six inches off the floor, so that the weight is entirely on the hands and toes. Keep the whole body straight and try to hold this position for ten to thirty seconds.

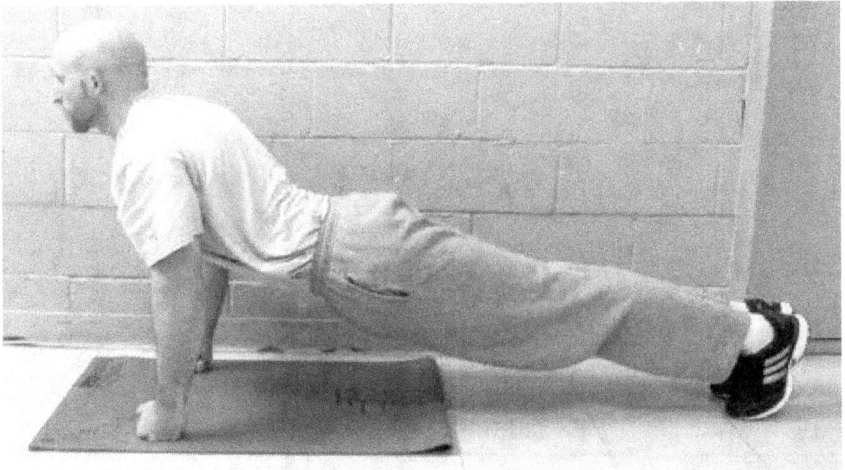

Knuckle push-up stand-Strengthens the arms, wrists and tones the abdomen and will release tension between the shoulder blades. Make a fist with your hands and place both knuckles on the floor, get into the push-up position. Flex your abs and keep your body very straight, try to keep this position for one minute, gradually working it up to five minutes.

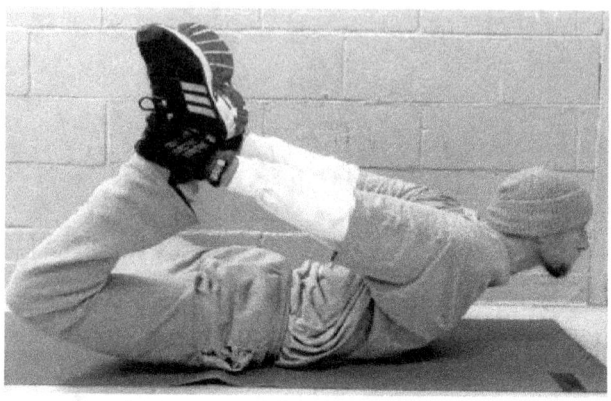

Bow Pose -
Makes the spine flexible, relieves back stress and tones abdominal organs.

Lie face down on the floor. Bend both knees and reach back with your hands to grasp the outer ankles. Lift your thighs as high as possible off the floor, while lifting your head and chest up as high as you can at the same time. Keep the arms straight and pull the shoulders back with the strength of the legs. Keep this position for five to fifteen seconds.

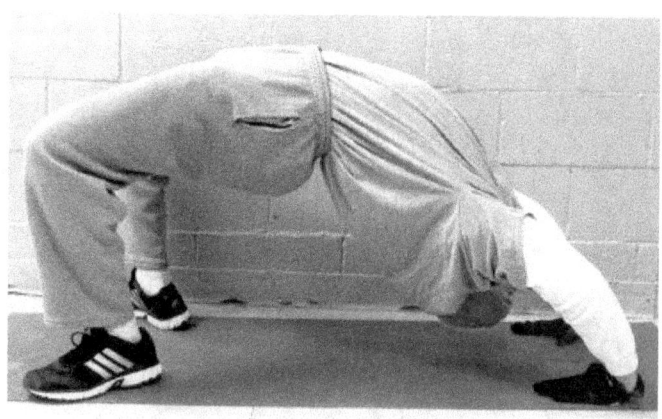

Bridge-
Strengthens the arms and wrists while giving the spine a maximum stretch. Lie on your back on the floor. Bend your knees and bring your heels up to your buttocks. Press the soles of your feet firmly against the floor. Bring the palms to the floor beside the shoulders, with the elbows pointing up. Then inhale and push the floor away with your palms and the soles of the feet, lifting up to an arch. Hold this position for five to fifteen seconds.

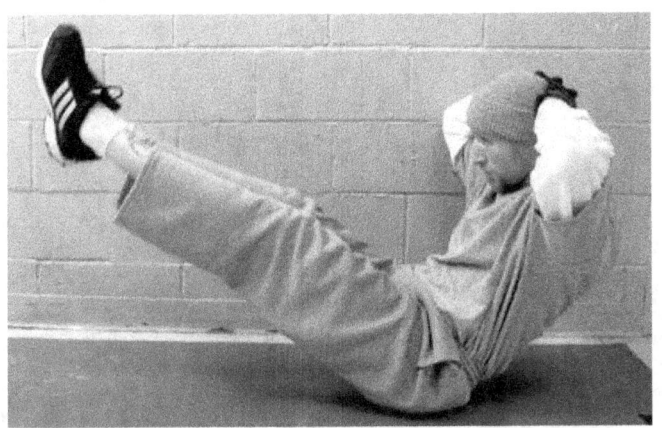

Boat Pose - Strengthens and tones the abdominal organs.
It also works the muscles of the lower back. Sit on the floor with your legs stretched out in front of you and the hands beside the hips on the floor.

Lean the body back slightly as you bend the knees and lift the legs off the floor. Bend the knees so your shins are parallel to the floor. Then slowly straighten the legs upward until they are extended. Keep your feet a bit higher than the head and try to interlace the fingers behind the head. Hold this position for five to ten seconds.

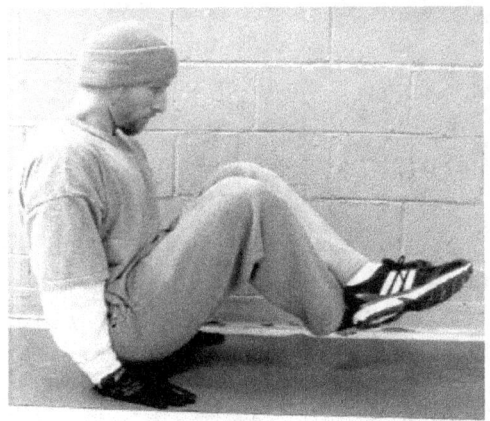

Scales Pose –
Strengthens the shoulders, arms and tones the abdomen.

Sit on the floor with legs crossed. Draw the knees close to your chest, and press your hands against the floor in front of the hips.

Lean forward and lift your butt and feet off the floor at the same time. Hold this position for five to ten seconds.

41

Head Stand- Strengthens the neck, shoulders, lower back, legs and makes the spine more flexible as well as developing balance.

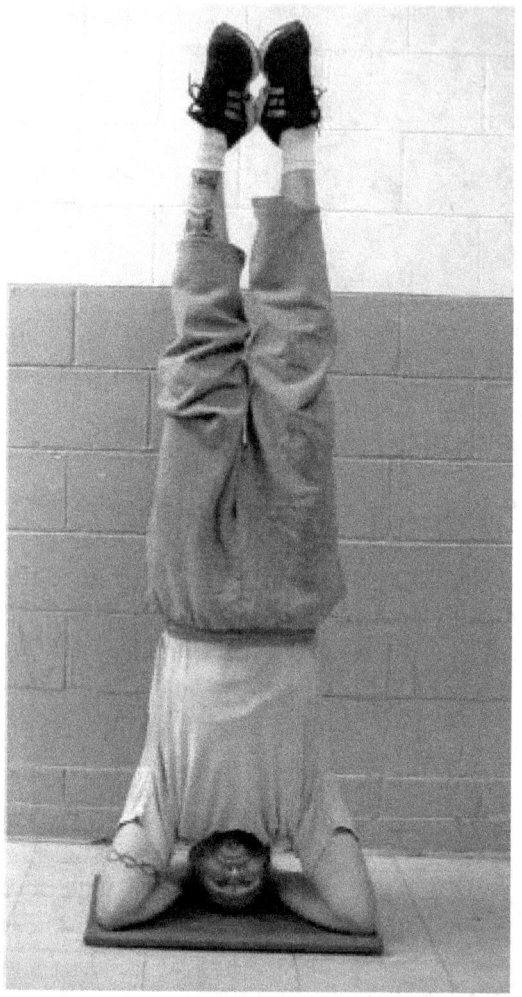

Place folded yoga mat or a blanket in front of you. Kneel in front of it. Put your forearms on the blanket with your elbows approximately at shoulder width and form a triangle by interlacing your fingers. Put the crown of the head between the wrists with the back of the head resting against the hands. Straighten your knees, bring your feet as close to the head as possible and slowly lift them off the floor. Lift your feet one by one and use the wall as a safeguard from falling in the beginning if necessary. Once the feet are lifted, straighten the legs, stretch the heels upward and keep your feet together. Hold this position for five to ten seconds and slowly build up your time by adding ten to twenty seconds each week until you reach five or even ten minutes.

Beginners Position

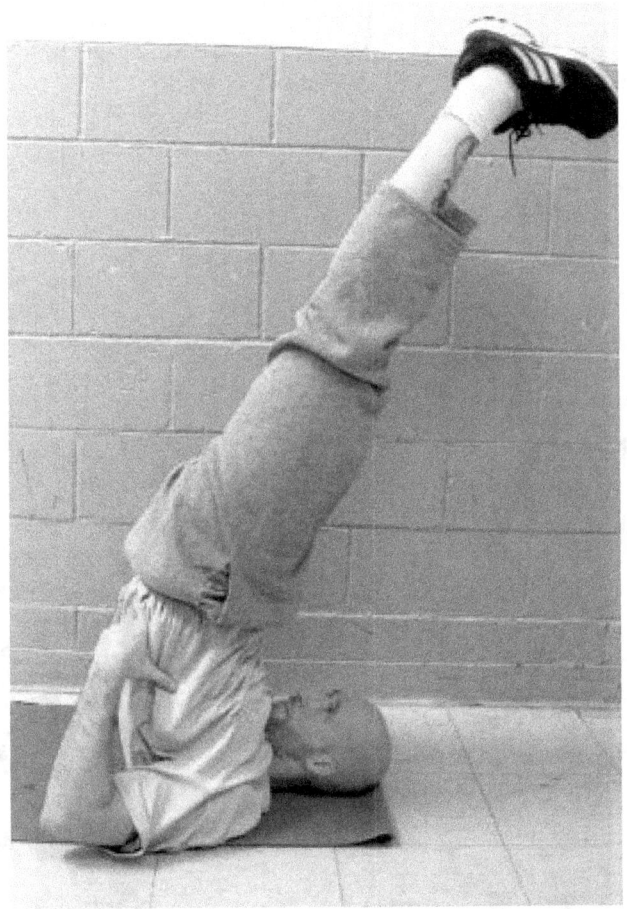

Shoulder Stand- Strengthens the neck, shoulders, legs and back.

Lie on your back over a folded blanket or a yoga mat. Bend your knees and bring your legs overhead. Support your back with your hands. Then straighten your legs in the air and stretch out your toes. Hold this position for twenty seconds and slowly build up your time to five or ten minutes.

Intermediate Shoulder Stand   Advanced Shoulder Stand

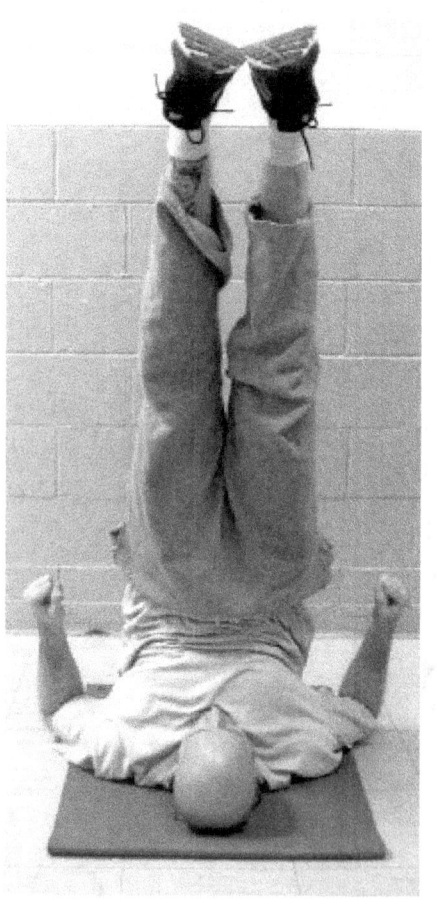

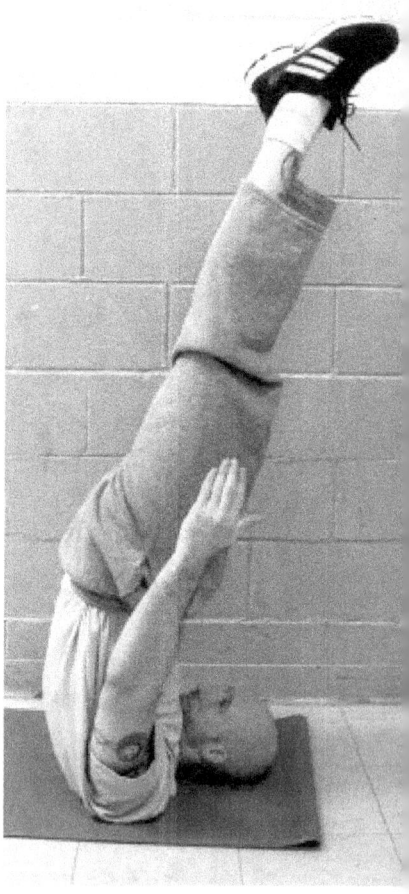

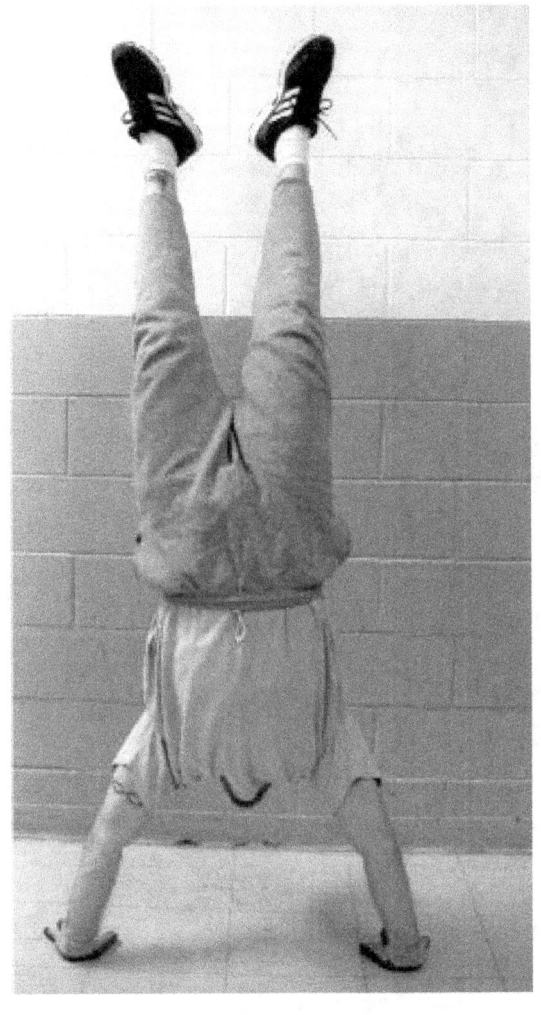

Hand Stand -

Strengthens the shoulders, arms, wrists, back and legs. Also develops great balance.

Fold forward from the hips and place your hands flat on the floor six-seven inches away from the wall. Have your palms shoulder width apart and your hands in a symmetrical position.

Walk forward until your shoulders are over your fingertips. Once you are on your tip toes it's time to kick up. Decide which will be your "kicking" leg. Keep the other leg bent with the heel near your buttock.

Bend your "kicking" leg and kick it up as your other leg swings up, reaching for the wall with the heel.

Then bring the feet together and stretch the heels up. Grip the floor with the fingers, straighten your arms and look a little forward of your hands. Hold this position for five to ten seconds. Gradually learn to hold this pose without the wall and try the posture away from the wall.

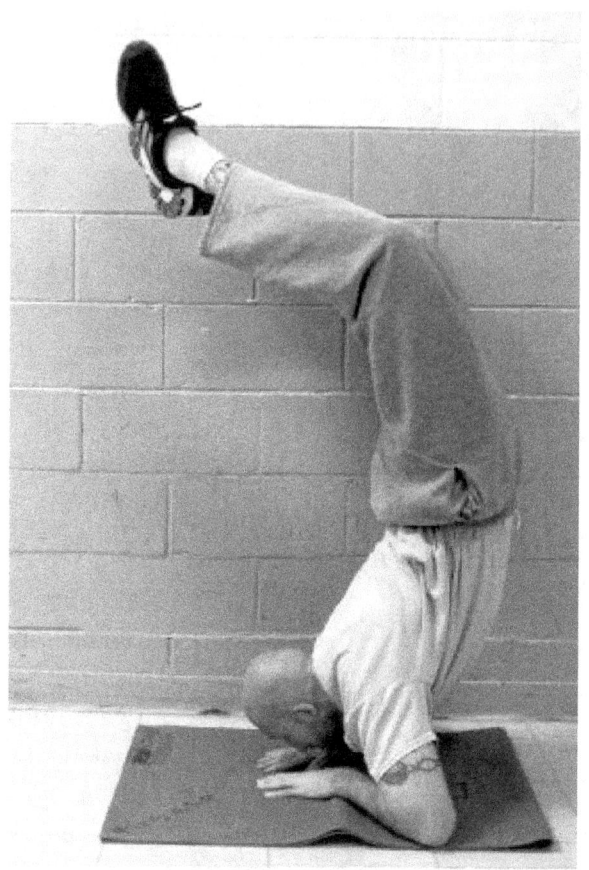

Elbow Balance- Strengthens the shoulders, arms and stretches the abdomen.

Place a yoga mat or a blanket in front of you. Kneel in front of it. Place your forearms on the blanket with your elbows shoulder width apart, the forearms parallel and the hands flat on the floor. Walk your feet toward the arms slowly bringing the weight of the body onto the elbows, then swing the legs up one by one, keeping them straight (when beginning, practice close to the wall). Bring the feet together and stretch the heels upward. Hold this position for five to ten seconds.

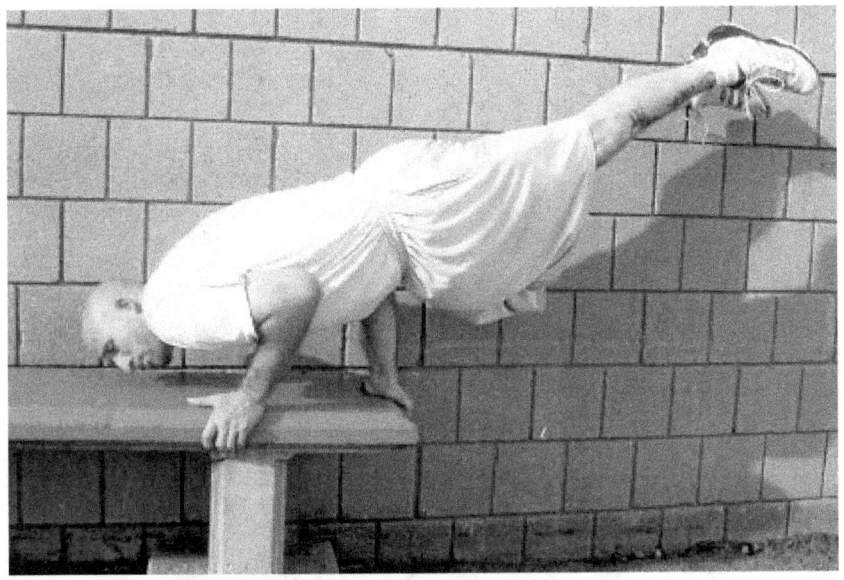

Elbow Lever-Strengthens the shoulders, arms, legs wrists, back and the abdomen.

Also develops great balance. An elbow lever is performed by leveraging your body weight against one or both elbows while balancing on your hand(s) with your body stretched out horizontally and resting on your arms. You should start practicing on any raised object, such as the bench or the table. This will allow you to wrap your fingers around the side of the object than using a flat handed grip instead. To start, lean forward and place the hands on the raised surface in front of you, with the fingers pointing back toward you. Position your elbows right up against your hip bones. Stretch the legs straight back so the weight of the body is resting on the wrists. Slowly move forward to transfer the weight of the body onto the hands and lift the feet off the floor. Concentrate on squeezing your midsection tight as you lift up, because some of your elbows will wind up against your stomach. Lift the head and the legs to extend them away and keep your whole body straight. Hold this position for five to ten seconds.

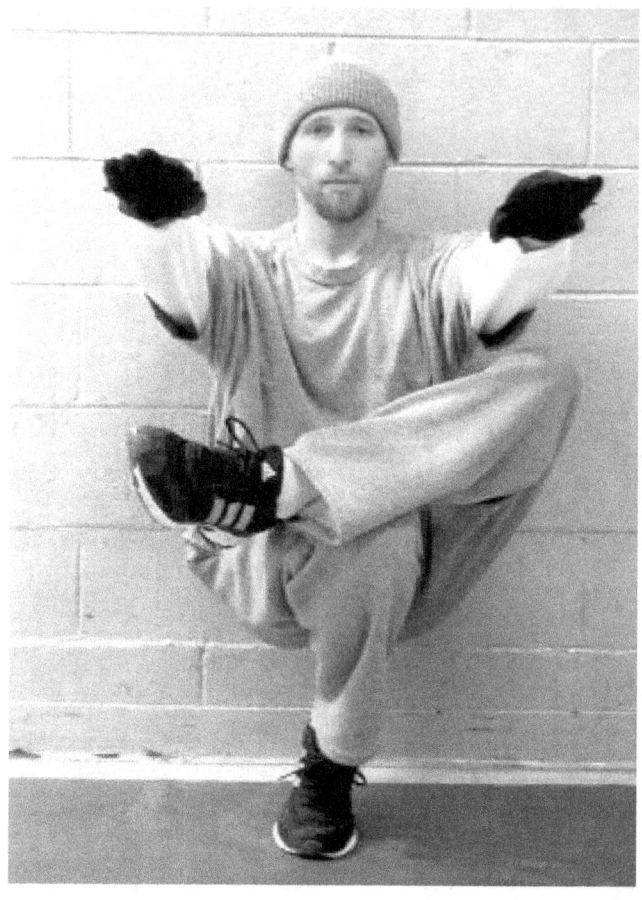

Toe Balance Pose-Strengthens the ankles, makes the hips flexible and develops balance.

Stand straight with your back against the wall. Lift the left heel up and rest it at the top of the right thigh. Using the wall for support, slowly sink down into a one-legged squat. If needed, use your fingertips on the floor for help, as you balance on the ball of your foot. Hold this position for five to ten seconds, then switch legs. Once you get more advanced, try to hold this position without the wall.

Abbs

Abbs training is also a part of core exercises. Which can improve your sports performance as well as offering general conditioning benefits. Yes, I like to have a good looking six pack, just like the next guy, but forget about looks for a second. Abdominals are more than a barometer of conditioning, they're a shield. Between the ribs and the hips lies nothing but flesh to protect vulnerable organs from a potential barrage of blows and injuries. So for me in particular, and the rest of the martial arts world, hard strong abbs can make a big difference.

However, the majority of people don't need to go an extra mile and basically by using your own body weight as resistance, and working to failure, for example, will help you get a flat lean mid-section. This will allow your waist to appear smaller as well. Remember one thing, abbs are made by hard work, but are exposed in the kitchen. Knowing your abdominal training will allow you to concentrate on specific muscle groups if needed.

Overal Abbs- Even though you can't completely isolate any single portion of your abdominals, you can involve a particular section over another through exercise selection. Attacking your abbs with all sorts of moves means that you're sure to cover the bases for a balanced mid-section.

Upper Abbs- When you bring your torso toward your legs you target your upper abbs. And, because you're naturally stronger during these moves, adding weight can make a big difference in the way your abbs pop. If you want your abbs to show deeper cuts, adding weight is one of your best bets.

Lower Abbs- The lower abbs are the weakest link along the chain of abdominal muscles. The key to targeting your lower abbs is to bring your legs toward your torso as with reverse crunches and hanging leg raises. If your lower abbs are a weakness, try doing them first in your ab routine and increase the frequency of these workouts throughout the month.

Inner Core - While all of these muscles I mentioned make up the overall core, here I specifically talk about the innermost abdominal muscles. You can think of the transverse abdominis as an internal weight belt, helping to provide stability to your spine by producing intra-abdominal pressure. This pressure, much like that provided by a weight belt, helps keep the spine in safe alignment during bent-over and squatting moves, protecting you from injury caused by the spine traveling forward toward the navel.

Obliques - Helping to complete the abdominal package are the internal and external obliques, which are responsible for trunk rotation and lateral flexion of the torso. Strong obliques are also integral to athletic performance, no matter what the genre. If you've neglected your obliques, the imbalance will be detected immediately when you begin these exercises. A dedicated approach will help bring balance to your mid-section.

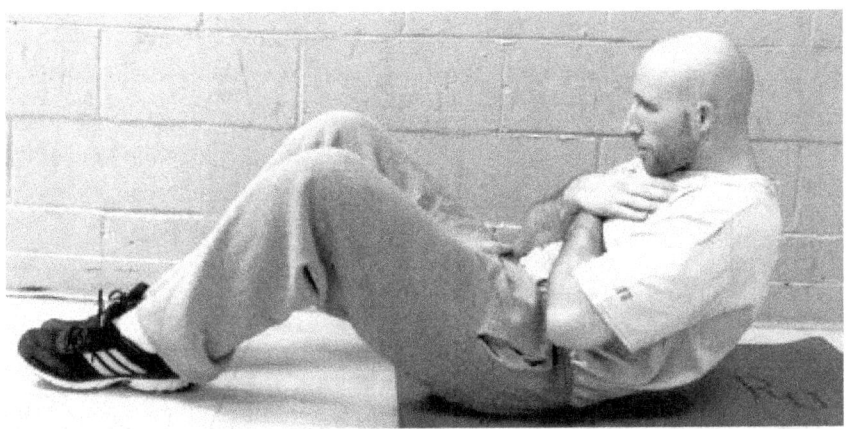

Crunch - Lie on your back with your knees bent and feet flat on the floor. Place your fingertips behind your ears. Now raise only your head and shoulders as you crunch your rib cage toward your pelvis. Return to the starting position and repeat quickly.

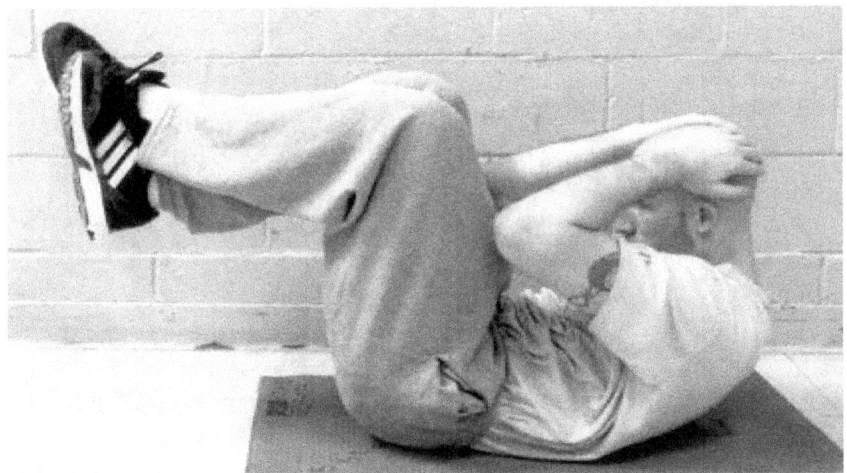

Double Crunch -
Lie on your back with your feet together and legs extended, holding them about six inches above the floor. Support your head lightly with your hands. Crunch upward and bring your knees toward your chest simultaneously. Return to the starting position and repeat.

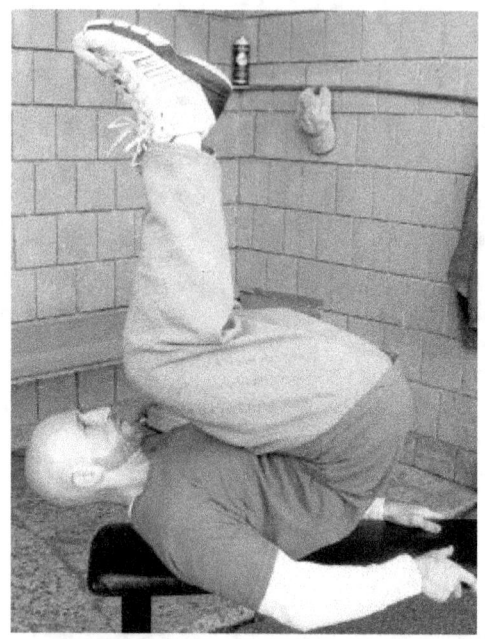

Reverse Crunch –
Lie on your back with your hands extended at your sides. Bend your knees at a ninety-degree angle, with your shins parallel to the floor.

Slowly bring your knees toward your chest, lifting your hips and glutes off the ground. Maintain the bend in your knees throughout the movement.

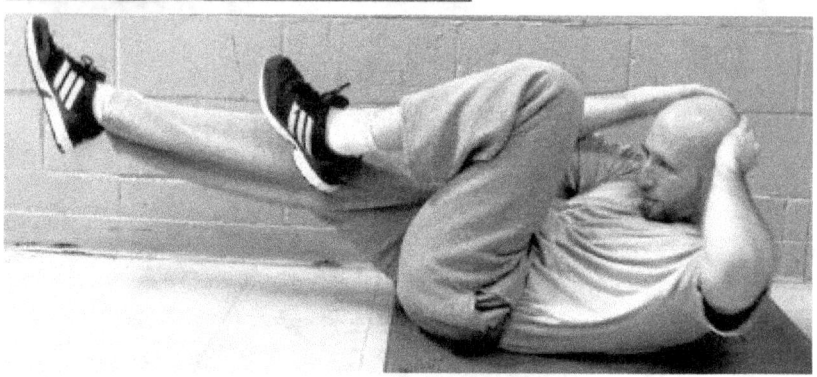

Bicycles - Lie on your back with your legs straight and your hands under your head. Hold one leg straight about six inches off the ground. Pull the knee of your other leg in toward your chest and touch it with the opposite elbow. Start riding, in other words, twist and turn back and forth, bringing your opposite elbow to your opposite knee in a slow movement. Be sure to extend each leg fully before bringing it back to your knee.

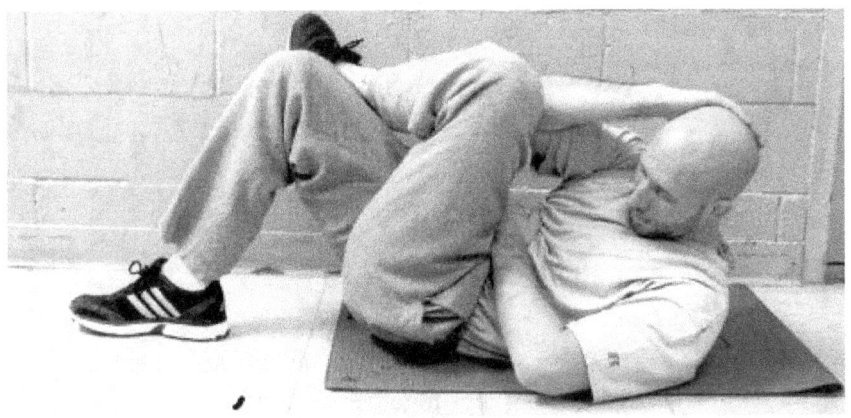

Cross Leg Crunch- Lie on your back with your knees bent and your right leg crossed over your left. Place the fingertips of your hand behind your head. As you crunch upward try to touch your right knee with your left elbow. Return to the starting position and repeat. Then switch legs and repeat the exercise to the opposite side,

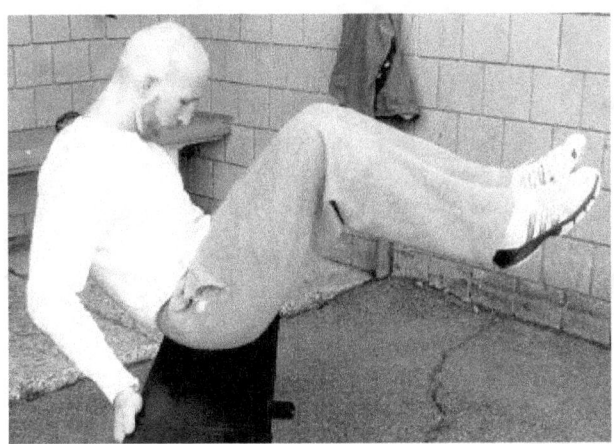

V-Ups-
Lie on your back, arms to your sides. Keep only your butt on the floor and bring your chest and your knees up toward each other as close as possible. Then lean your chest back and straighten your legs out so that both your shoulders and feet are only few inches from the floor.

53

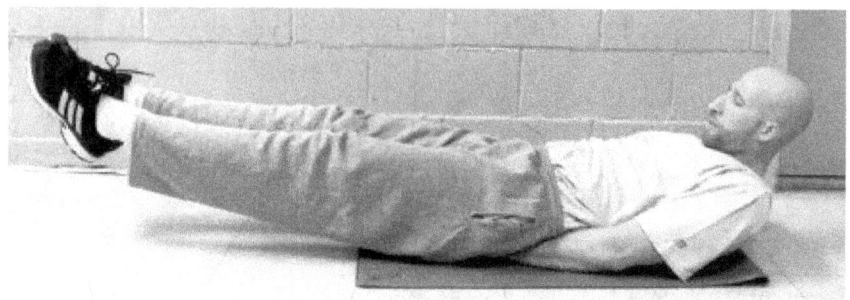

Vertical Scissors- Lie on your back with your hands under your butt and your head up. Keep your legs together and straight, six inches from the floor. Raise your right leg up to three feet in the air, and then bring it back down as you raise your left leg. This can be done fast or slow as long as you keep the motion very controlled.

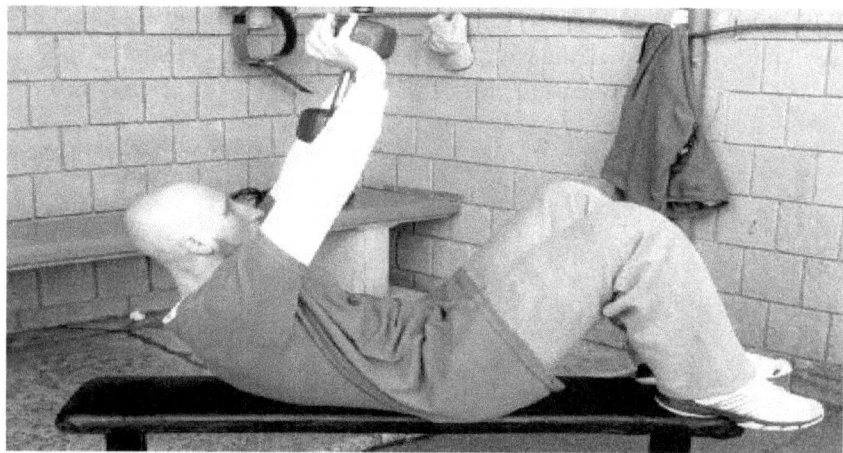

Weighted Crunch- Lie on your back with your knees bent and feet flat on the floor. Hold a dumbell with two hands above your chest and keep your arms straight. Now raise only your head and shoulders as you crunch your rib cage toward your pelvis. Hold this position for a second before lowering back to the starting position. Your arms should reach full extension when you touch the floor. Contract your abs to reverse the motion bringing the weight back to your chest at the top.

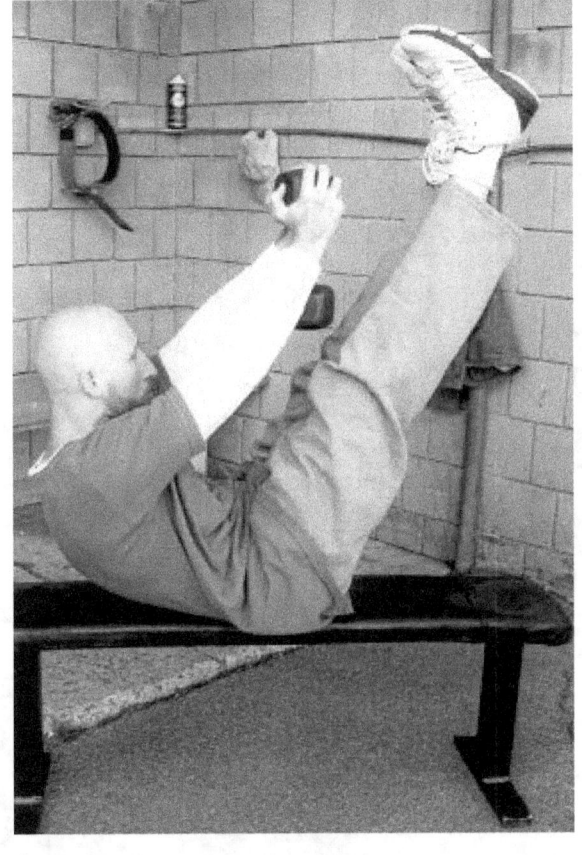

Weighted V-Sit –
Lie on your back with your legs together and hold a dumbell over your chest with both hands and keep your arms straight.

Lower the weight in an arc overhead toward the floor behind you and lift your legs six to eight inches off the floor.

Press your lower back into the floor and flex your feet.

Now, simultaneously bring your legs and torso together while keeping your arms extended over your head. Your goal is to form a V-shape with your upper and lower body, with your abbs serving as the base of the V.

Slowly lower back to the starting position and repeat.

Hanging Knee Raise – Grab onto a pull-up bar and hang.

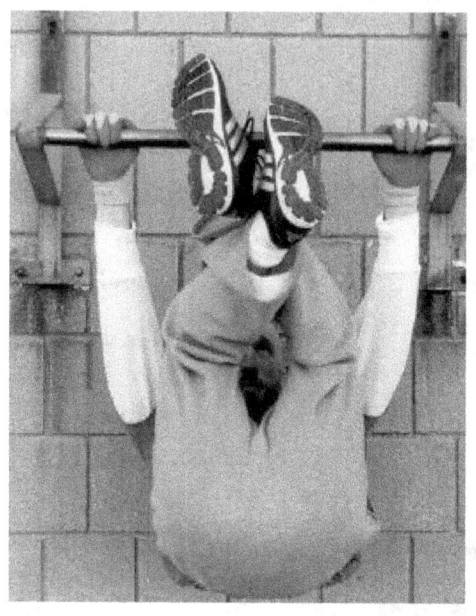

Now, pull your knees into your core, curling your tailbone under a bit to emphasize a contraction in your abbs.

Lower your legs without allowing your body to swing, and repeat motion.

Hanging Leg Raise – Grab onto a pull-up bar and hang.

Now raise your legs up to your chest, rounding your back so your feet touch the bar.

Lower your legs as slowly as you can control and repeat motion,

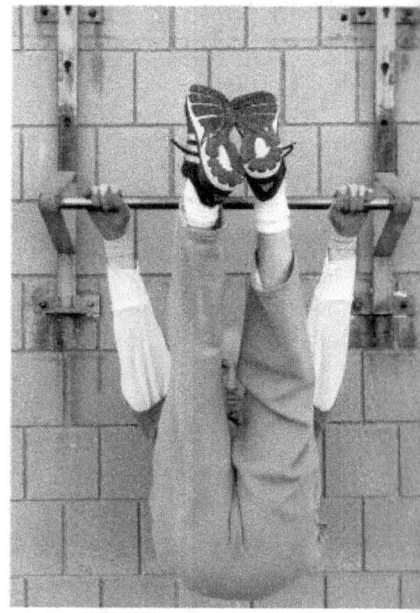

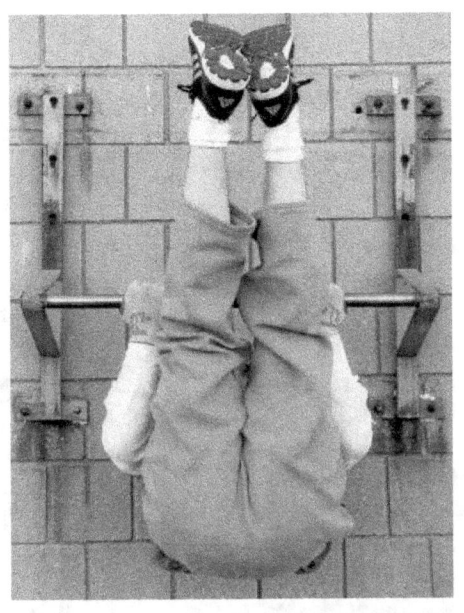

Windshield Wipers –
Grab onto a pull-up bar and hang. Now raise your legs up to your chest, rounding your back so your feet touch the bar and twist your legs from side to side like the windshield wipers of a car. You can think of it as only the top half of the circle.

Go slow when performing these movements and focus on good form, rather than how many reps you can perform.

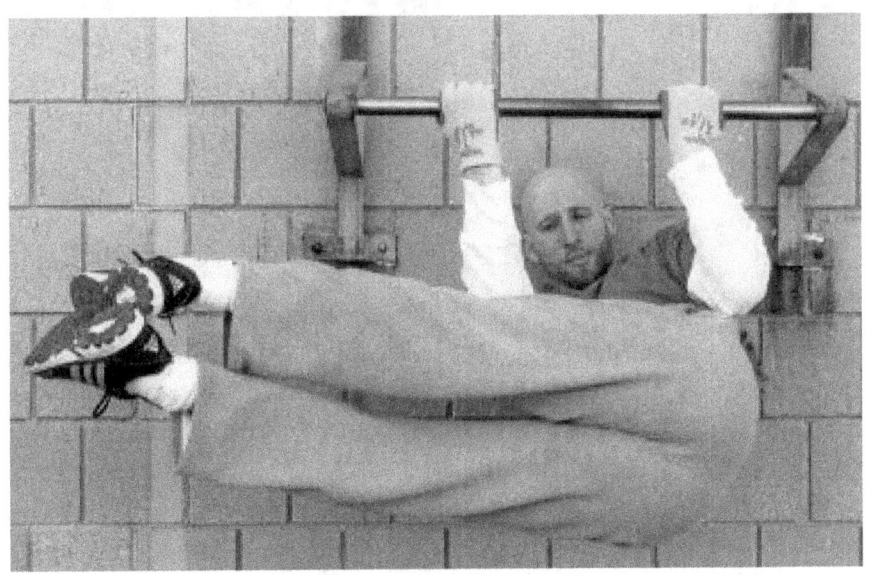

Step 1

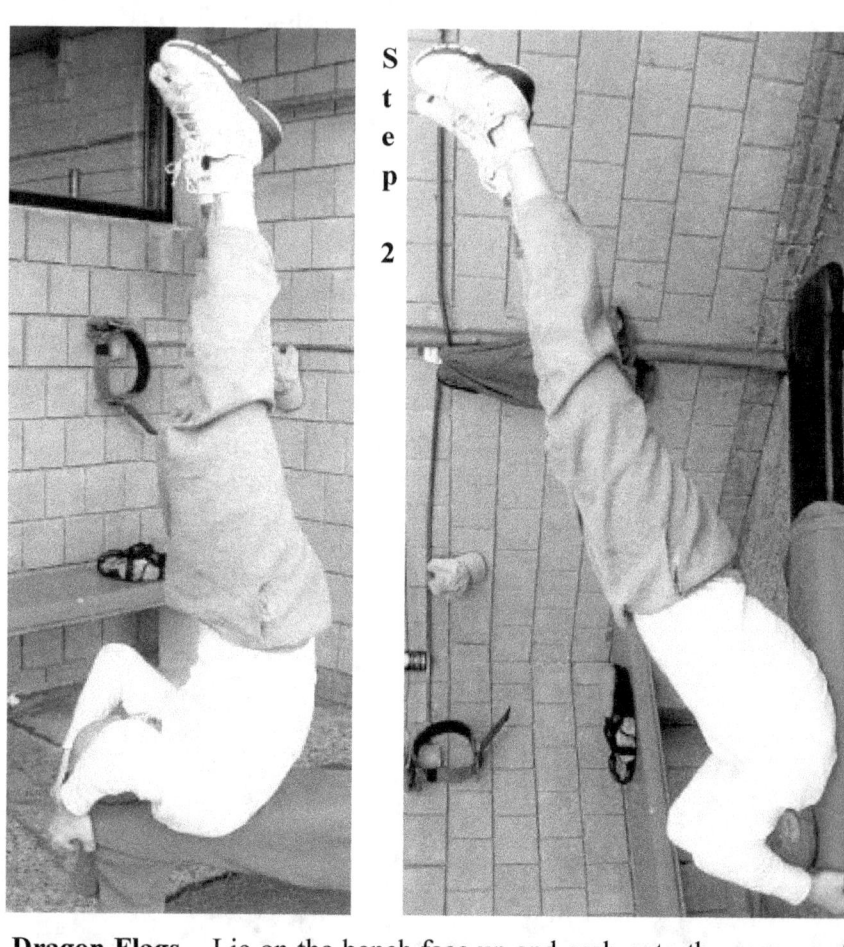

Dragon Flags – Lie on the bench face up and grab onto the corners of the bench above your head. Basically you are performing a lying leg raise in which you lift your hips and lower back off the bench until your body is perpendicular to the floor. Raise and lower yourself slowly making this function as a plank. At the end of your last rep, lower your whole body six to eight inches away from the bench and hold this position for as long as you can. (Kind of like Rocky, in the movie, "Rocky IV") So let's call it "Rocky Flag."

Legs

Pretty often too much attention is devoted to building the muscles above the waist, but you cannot forget leg training. Not only do strong legs complement a strong upper body, but legs are the driving force of our entire body. Having powerful legs makes everything else you do, from walking up the stairs to carrying heavy loads, easier. Not training the legs will hold back your gains in every department. This being factual because they are enormous muscles, working the legs causes greater release of natural anabolic hormones than any other body part. This contributes to the growth of all your muscles over time. So make sure you include a leg training routine in your weekly schedule.

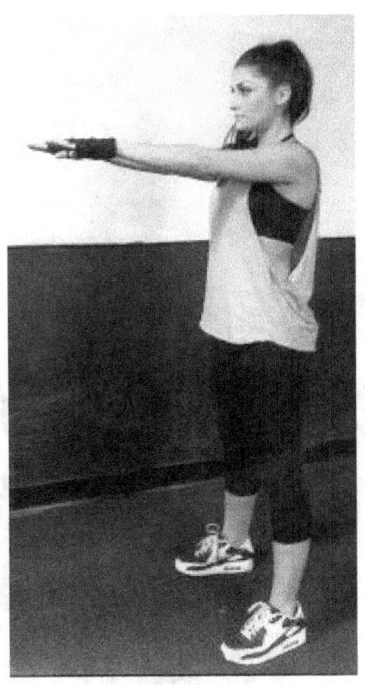

Squats –
(A great simple exercise to strengthen all sorts of muscles in the lower body, especially legs.) Stand with your feet shoulder width apart. Maintain a straight back as you perform the exercises.

With your head up and eyes forward, bend your knees as you slowly lower yourself into a squatting position. You can either stretch your arms out ahead of you or put your hands behind your ears.

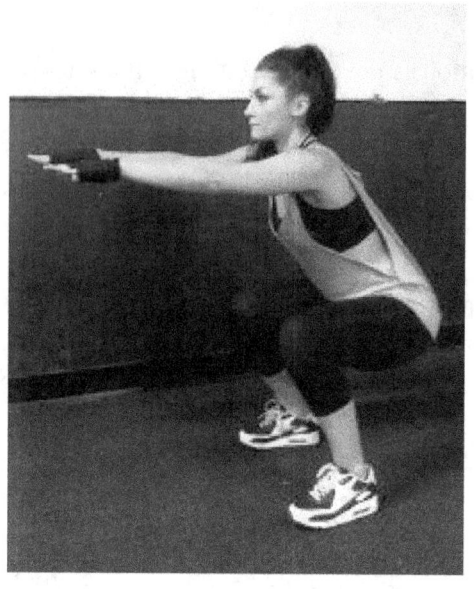

Squats -

Lower your body to a position where your thighs are almost parallel to the floor. Return to the starting position and repeat.

Goblet Squat-

Stand with your feet slightly beyond shoulder width.

Cup one end of a dumbell with both hands and hold it vertically in front of your chest, with your elbows pointing down. Keeping the natural arch in your back, push your hips back, bend your knees and squat.

Pause and push yourself back up to a standing position and repeat.

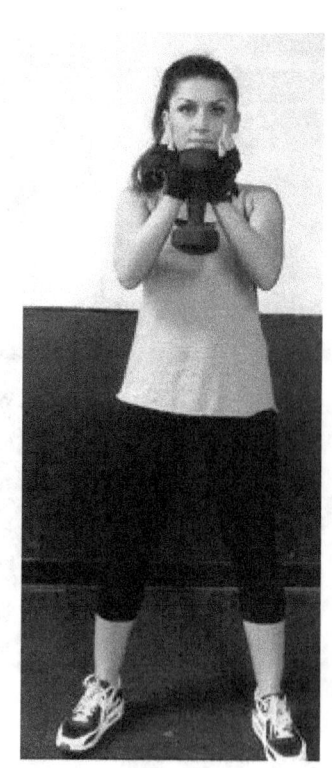

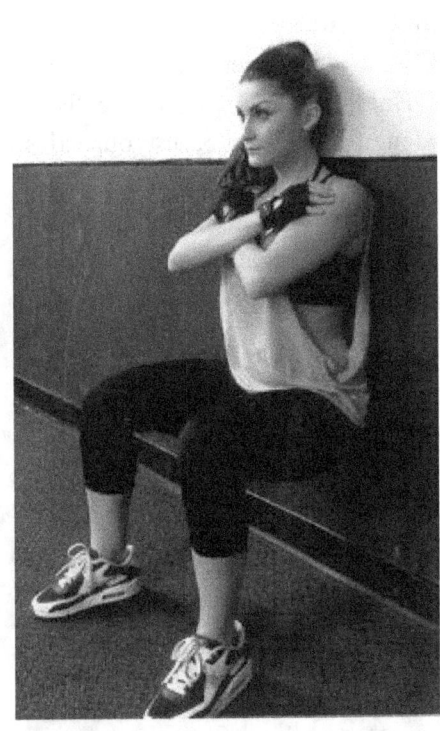

Invisible Chair Squat-

Stand with your back to a wall. Move your feet away from the wall, but keep your hips and back against the wall for support. Bending at the knees, lower your body until your thighs are parallel to the floor and knees bent at ninety degrees. Hold this position for as long as you can, if it gets too easy, try holding some additional weight in your hands above the thighs.

Invisible Chair Squat –
With Weights

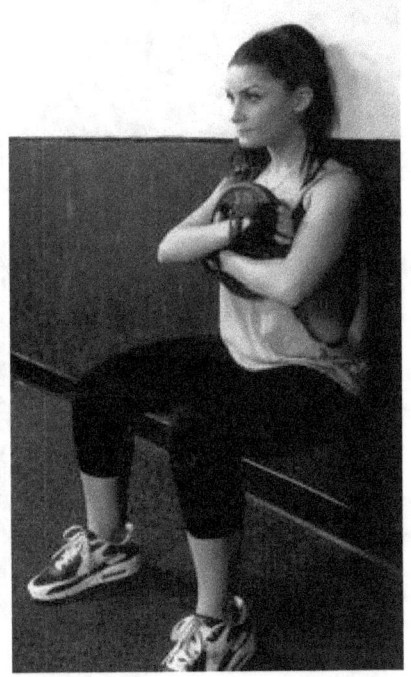

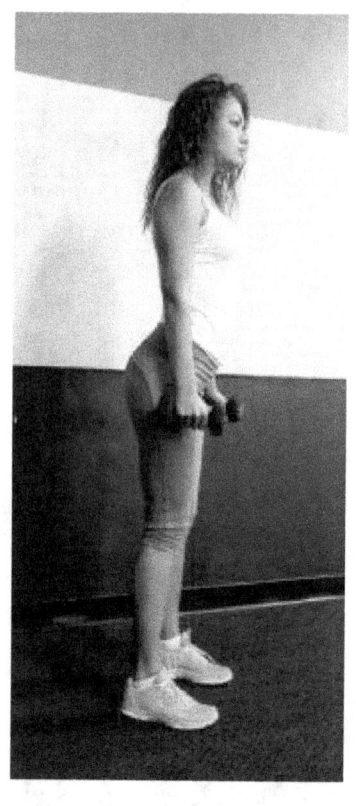

Dumbell Squat -

Stand with your feet shoulder width apart. Holding a pair of dumbells at arm's length directly next to your sides, (palms in). Maintain a straight back, bend your knees, and slowly lower yourself into a squat. Pause and push yourself back up to a standing position and repeat.

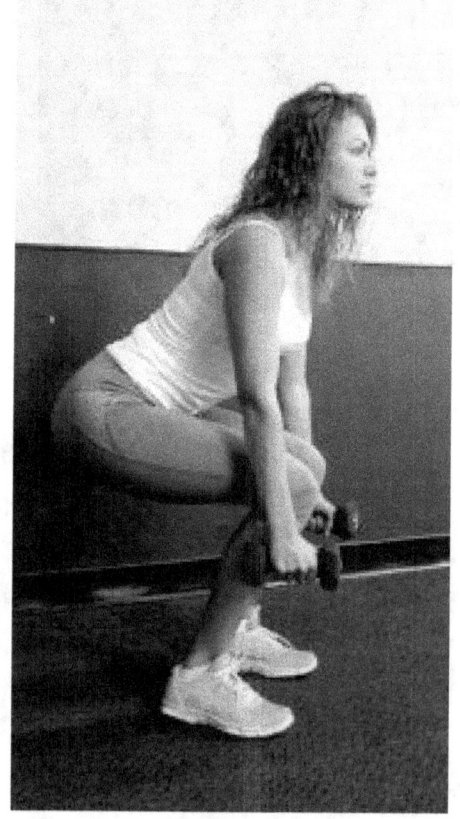

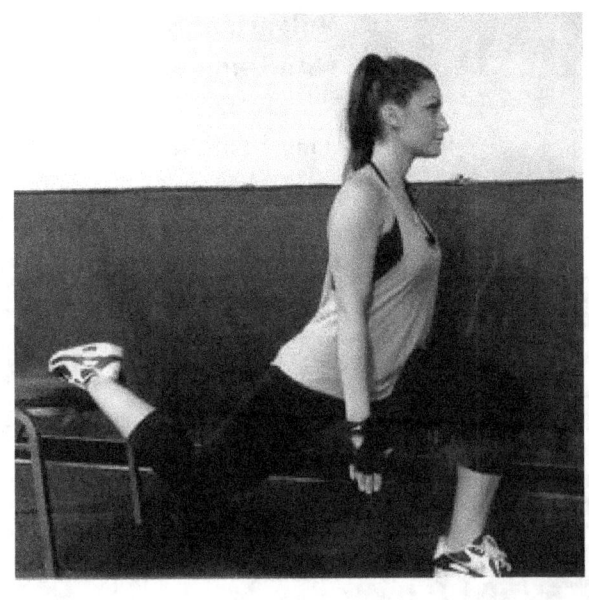

Bulgarian Split Squat -
Stand tall with your hands at your sides. Place the top of one foot on a bench or a chair about two feet behind you. Lower your body as far as you can into a squat. Pause, and push yourself back up to a standing position and repeat. Do the same number of repetitions on each side.

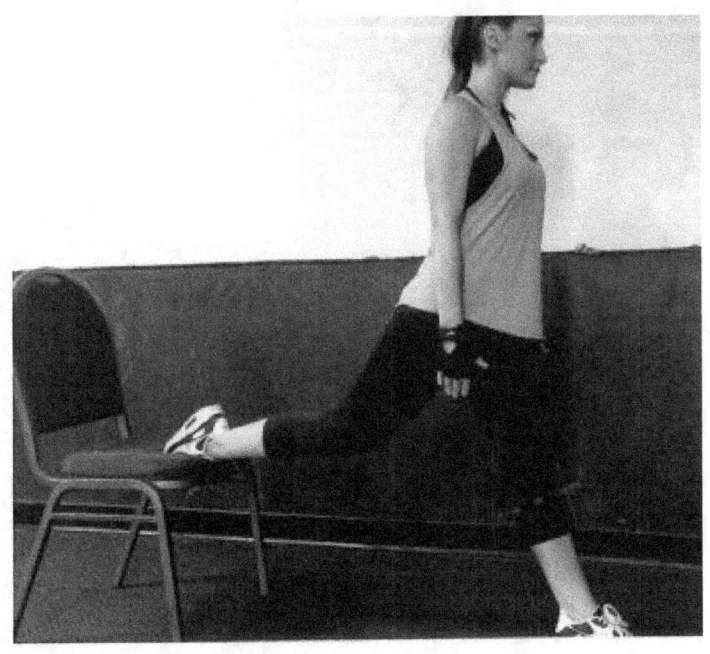

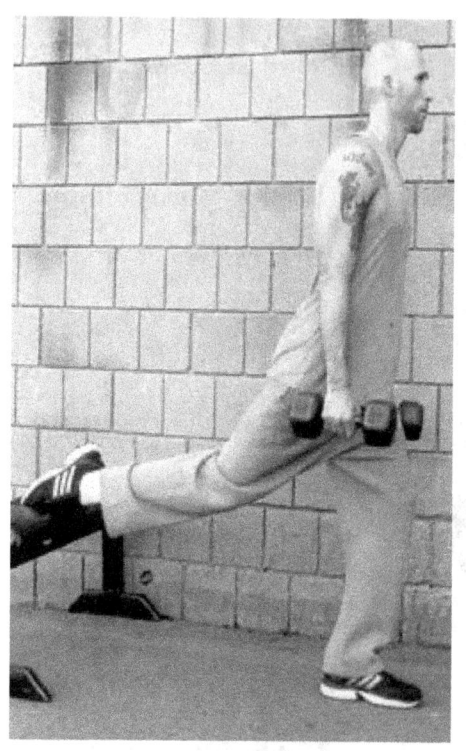

Bulgarian Split Squat with Dumbells –
Stand tall holding a dumbell in each hand.

With your arms hanging down at your sides. Place the top of one foot on a bench or chair behind you.

Slowly lower your body as far as you can. Pause, and push yourself back up to a standing position and repeat. Do the same number of reps on each side.

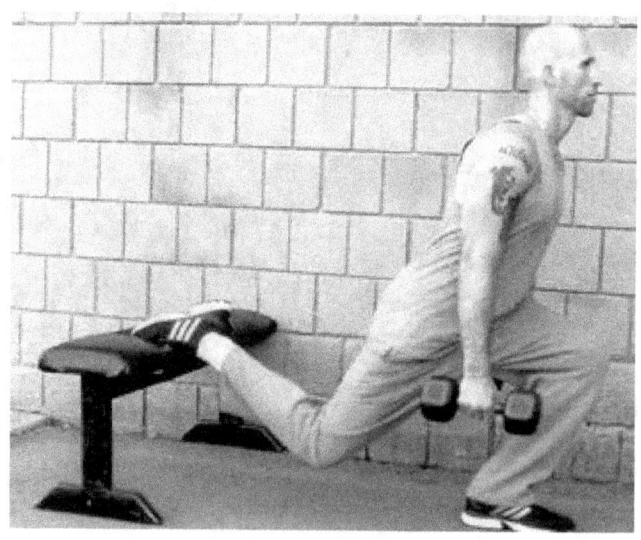

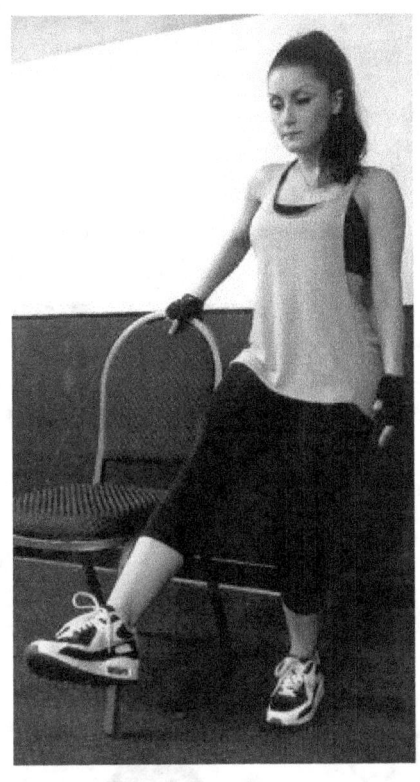

One Legged Squat -

Stand with your working leg next to a chair. Hold on to the chair with one arm as you extend your working leg out in front of you. Push your hips back and slowly lower your body as far as you can. Make sure your leg is doing the work your arm is just holding the chair for balance. Using only your working leg, push yourself back up and repeat. Do the same number of reps on each side.

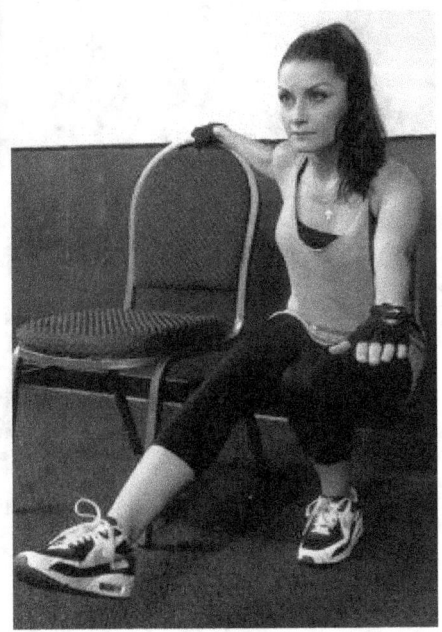

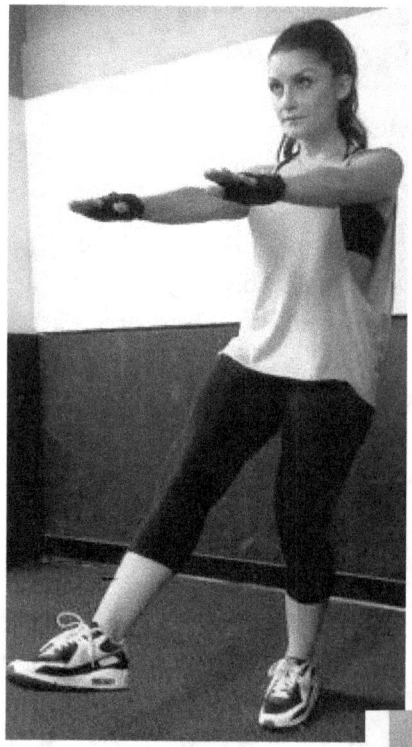

Pistol Squat -
Stand with your feet shoulder width apart. Raise one leg in front of you, parallel to the floor. Stretch your arms out ahead of you for balance, push your hips back and slowly lower your body as far as you can, then explode back up and repeat. Do the same number of reps on each side.

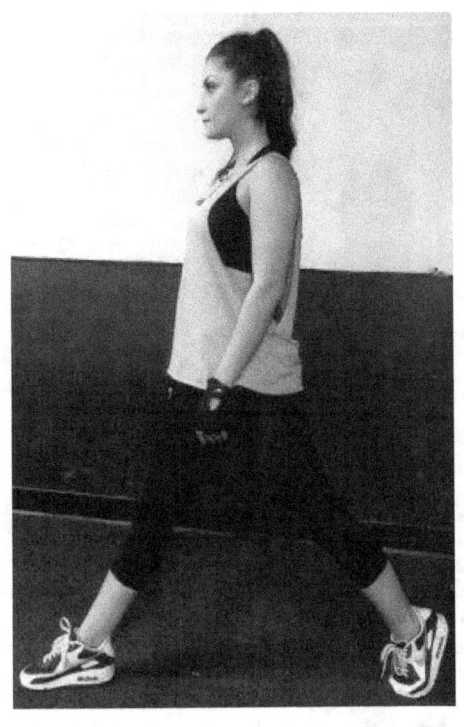

Lunge –

Stand tall, with your hands by your hips or behind your head. With your left foot, take a big step forward, bending your knees and lowering your hips until your right knee almost touches the floor. Keep your back straight throughout the exercise, then push up with your left leg and step back to the starting position. Do the same number of reps on each side.

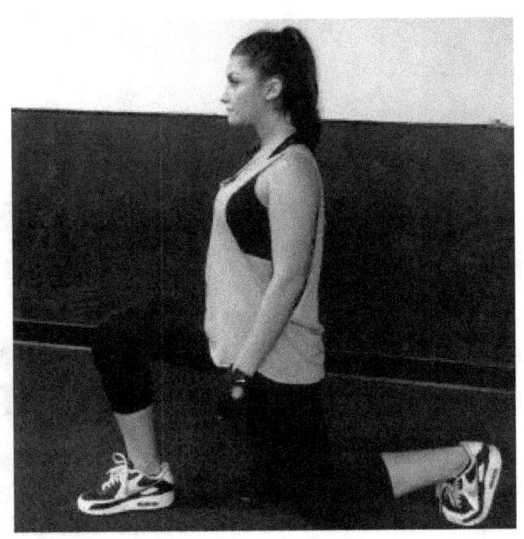

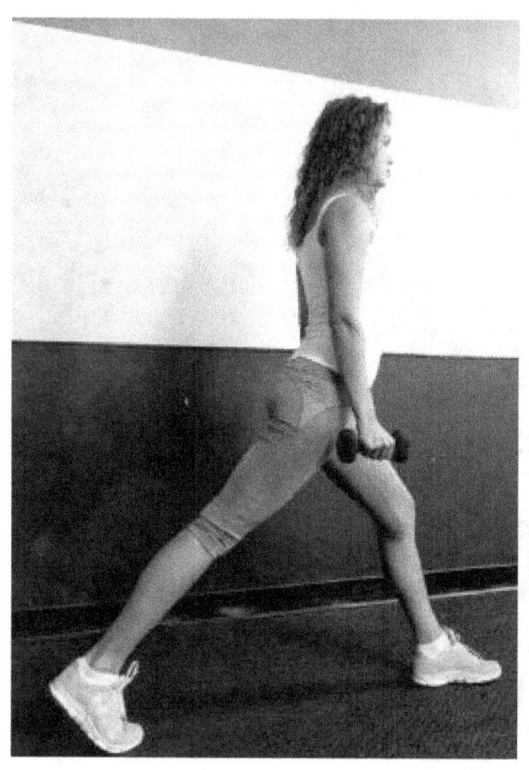

Dumbell Lunge -
Stand with your feet shoulder width apart, holding a dumbell in each hand, with your arms hanging down at your sides.

With your left foot, take a big step forward and lower yourself down until your left thigh is parallel to the floor. Push yourself back into the starting position and repeat the lunge, stepping forward with your right foot this time.

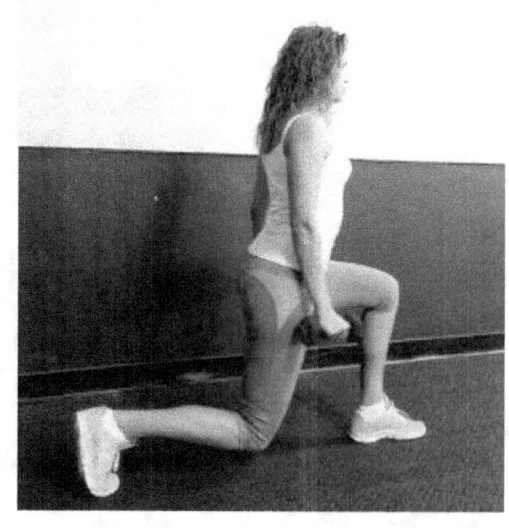

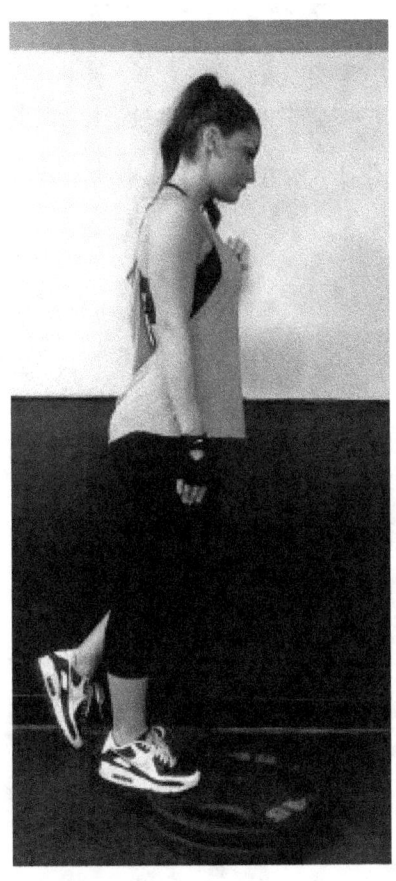 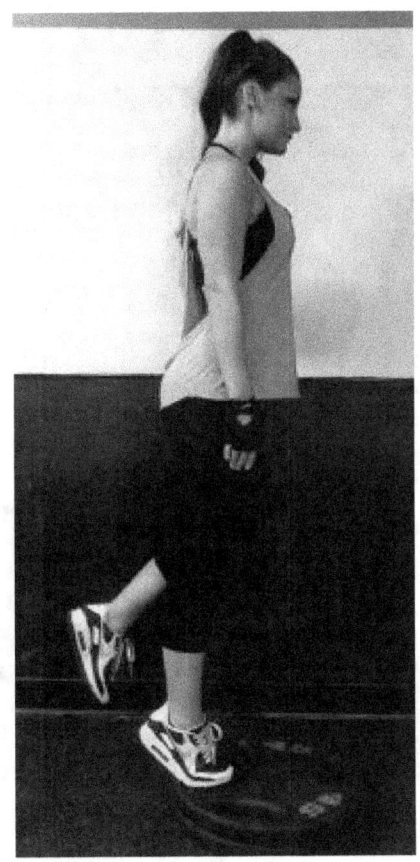

Calf Raises-

Stand on one leg on a box or another low level stable platform. Stand on the edge of the box, so your heel hangs off the edge. With your knee straight but not locked. Grab a hold of the wall for balance and lower your heel, sinking as far as possible. Come all the way up onto the ball of your feet and toes, lifting yourself as high as you can. Hold at the top for a count of one, then slowly lower all the way back to the starting position, sinking as deeply as you can down on your heel. Do the same number of reps on each side.

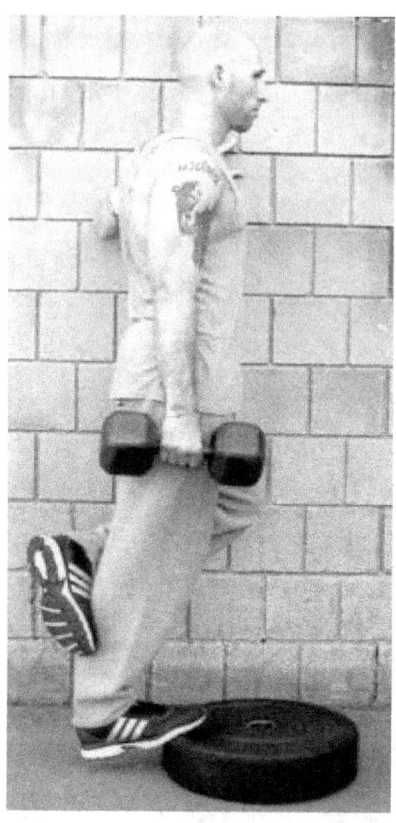 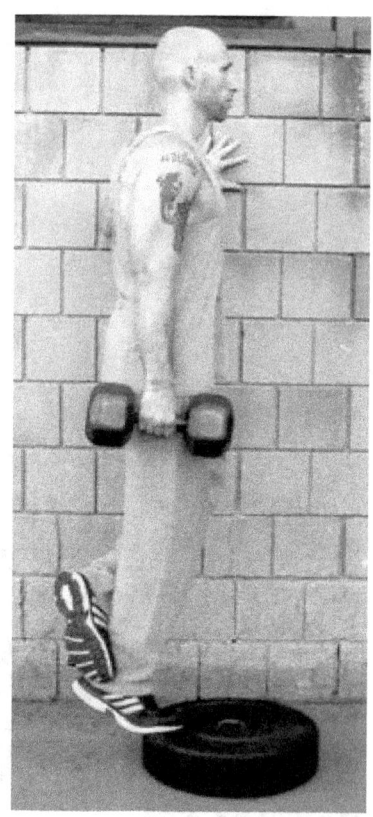

Dumbell Calf Raise-

Stand on the edge of the box with your right foot and grab a dumbell with your right hand. Keep your left hand on the wall for balance and lower your right heel as far as your calf will stretch. Hold this position for a second, and then push yourself up as high as you can onto the ball of your foot. Hold this position for one second and repeat. Do the same number of reps on each side.

You can also turn your toes slightly inward to concentrate on the outside of your calve muscle or turn your toes slightly outward to concentrate on the inside of your calve muscle.

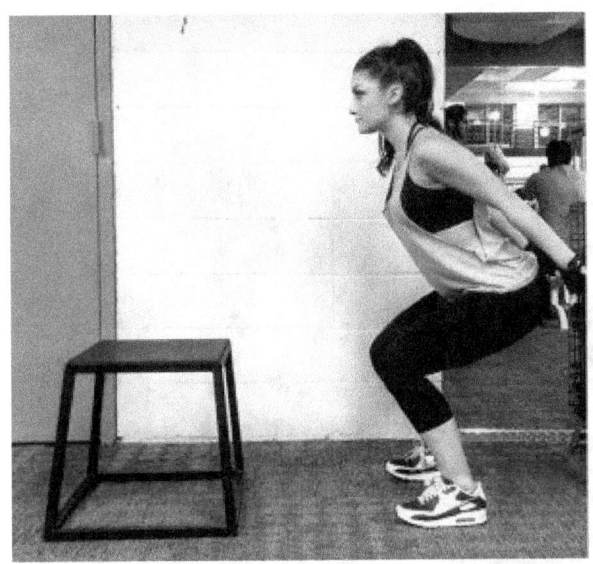

Box Jump - Stand facing a low box or a low adjustable bench. Your feet should be shoulder width apart, hands at your sides. Push your hips back, bend your knees and swing your arms back as you lower your body into a squat.

Then reverse the move as you swing your arms forward and explode forcefully onto the object, landing with both feet. Step down and repeat.

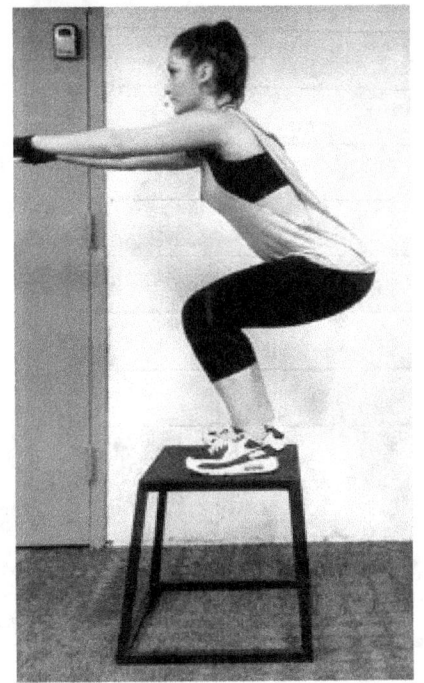

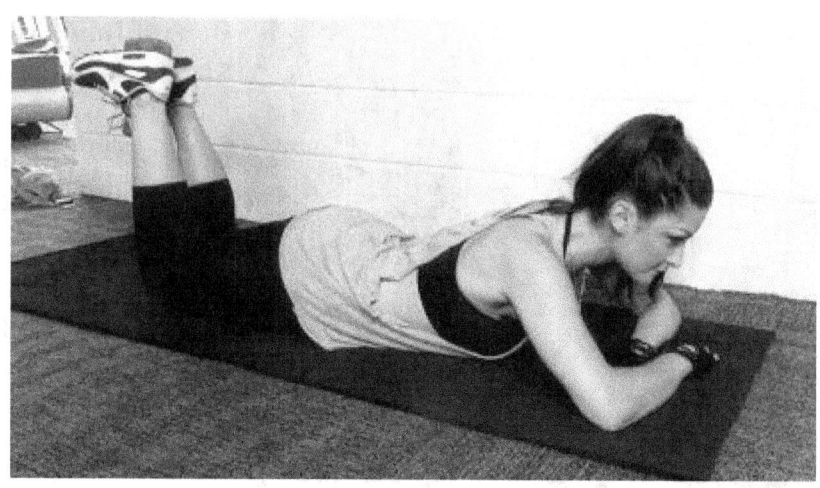

Glute/Hamstring Curl -

Lay on your stomach with elbows bent and hands in a comfortable position in front of your chest. Hold a dumbell between your feet and make sure your knees are bent at a ninety degree angle. Keeping your thighs and the entire upper body on the ground, uncurl your legs toward the floor until the weight nearly touches. Hold this position for a second and return to the starting position.

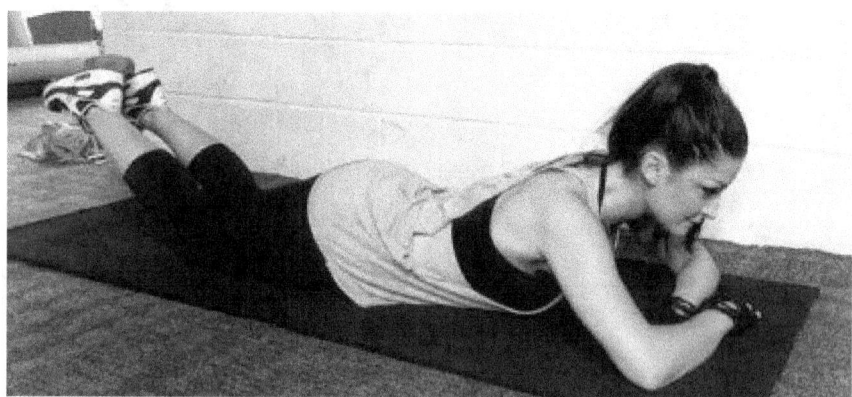

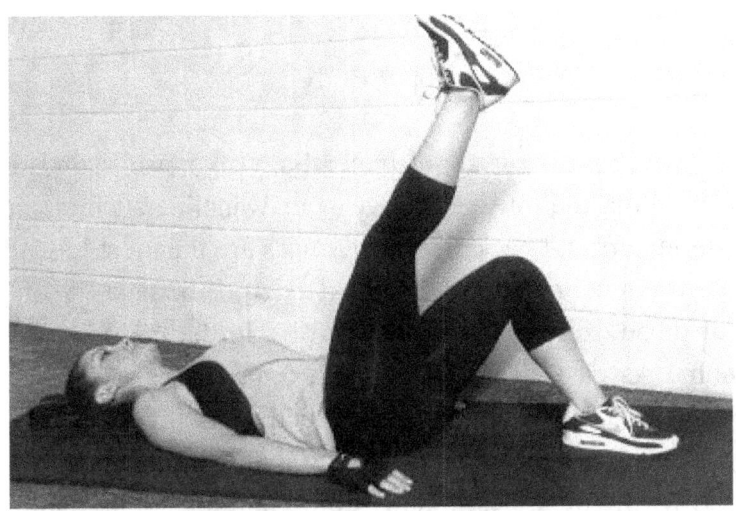

One Legged Hip Thrust - Lie face up on the floor and bend one leg so your foot is close to your butt, while the other remains extended. Extend your arms along your sides, palms down, then lift the extended leg straight up into the air perpendicular to the floor, keeping your hips square and your abs tight. Press down into your grounded heel and lift your hips toward the ceiling. Hold this position for a second and slowly lower back to the starting position.

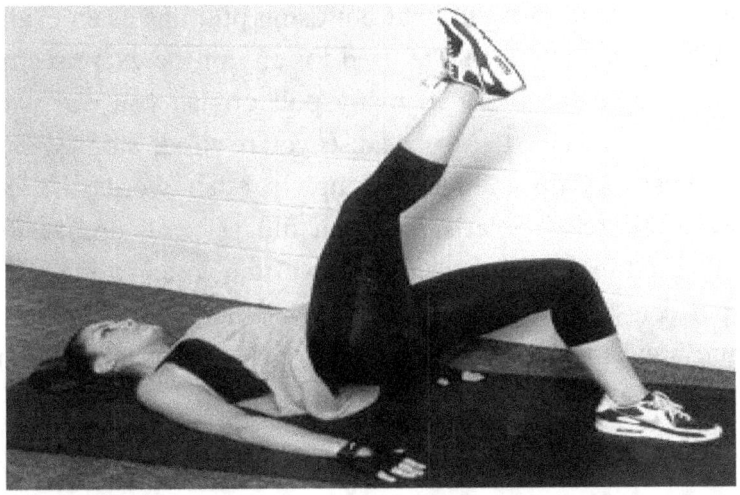

Upper Body

When we're talking about upper body exercise, it primarily means working the muscles above your waistline such as: arms, chest, shoulders and back. These exercises are the most rewarding because you tend to see results quickly. And believe it or not most of those exercises you can perform in the comfort of your own home. As easy as it may sound, upper body exercises are some of the easiest to perform incorrectly and that can cause an injury or you just fool yourself into believing you're making progress when you are essentially doing nothing at all. While this is the case with any exercise, it's very important that you take some time to learn the proper form or you will be wasting your time.

With every upper body exercise you also need to figure out how many times to do each. Obviously you won't get far if you do just two pull ups and call it a day, but how do you know how many pull ups and sets to do and when to take a break and so on? Here is a method to figure that out using pull ups as an example, (however this method can be used for any of the exercises in the upper body section). Do as many pull ups as you can without taking a break. Don't stop because you're tired, stop when you can't physically do another pull up. In other words, it's called "muscle failure". So let's say, you did six pull ups total that would result in the number three. Next time you do your pull ups, do four sets of that number (three for example) with about one minute breaks in between. If you can manage to do more on the last set, you should definitely rep out.

As you get stronger you'll need to increase the number of pull ups you do in each set. And if you ever notice things are getting too easy for you, just strap some weight to your body, like a ten to twenty pound book bag or pick up heavier dumbells with other upper body exercises.

Arms

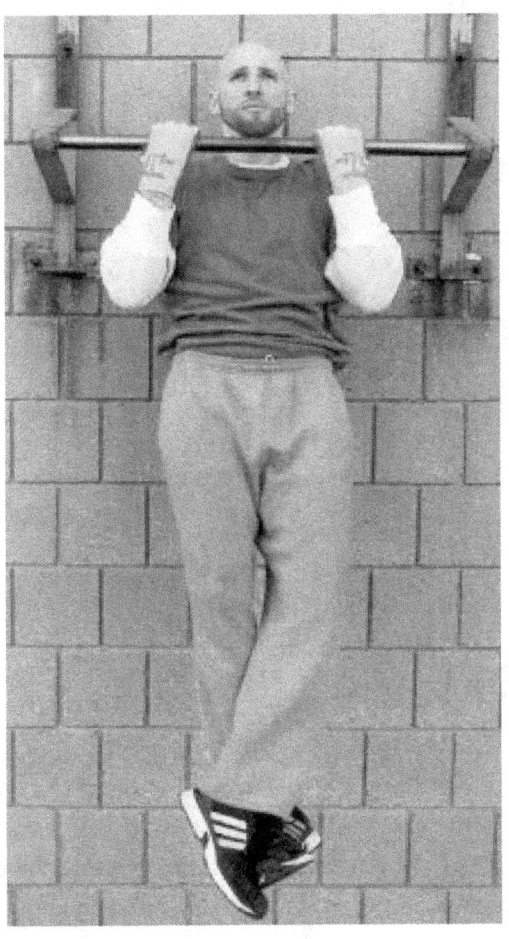

Chin up-
(Targets the biceps) Grasp the chin up bar under hand, slightly inside shoulder width, with your hand at arms length.

Cross your ankles behind you. Pull your chest to the bar, pause and return to a dead hang with your arms fully extended.

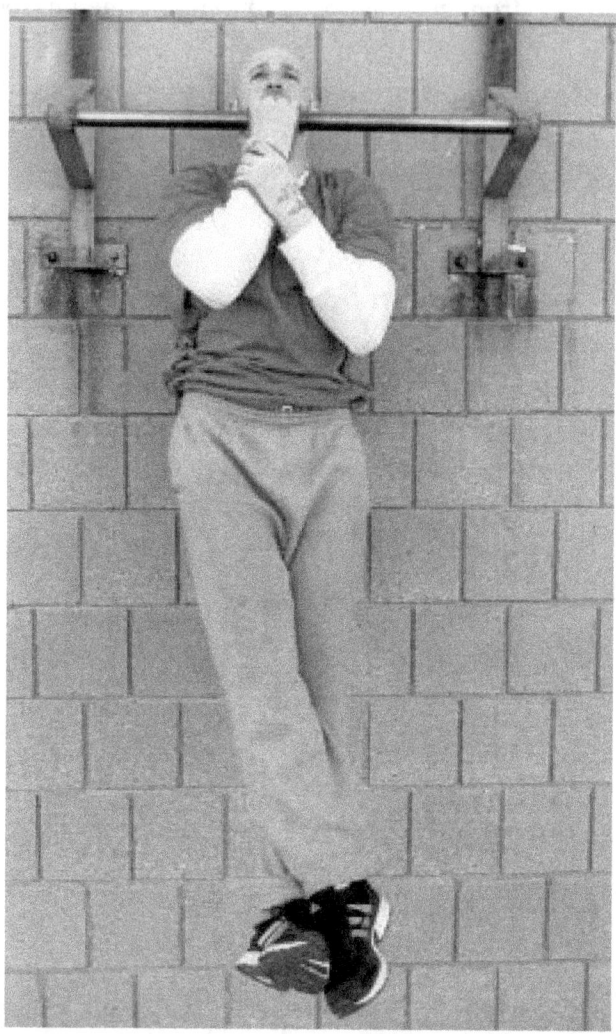

One Hand Chin up-

(Targets the biceps) Grasp the chin up bar under hand with your right hand. Grab your right forearm with the left hand. Cross your ankles behind you. Bring your chin to the bar, pause and slowly lower your body. Repeat the same amount of reps on the opposite side.

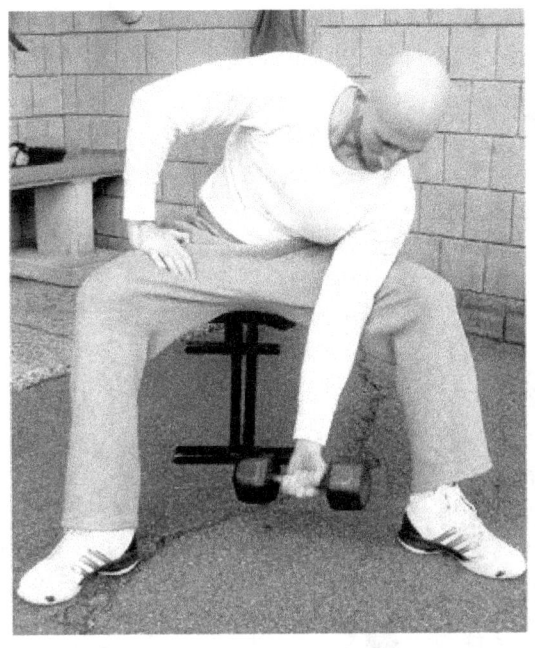

Seated Curl-
(Targets the biceps) Sit on a bench, legs apart, with the dumbell on the floor between your feet.

Pick up the weight and use your inner thigh as a support for your elbow and forearm and curl the weight.
Keep your elbow anchored against your inner thigh.

Keep the other hand on the opposite knee. Lower the weight with control. Move with a full range of motion before bringing the weight back up again. Repeat the same amount of reps on the opposite sides.

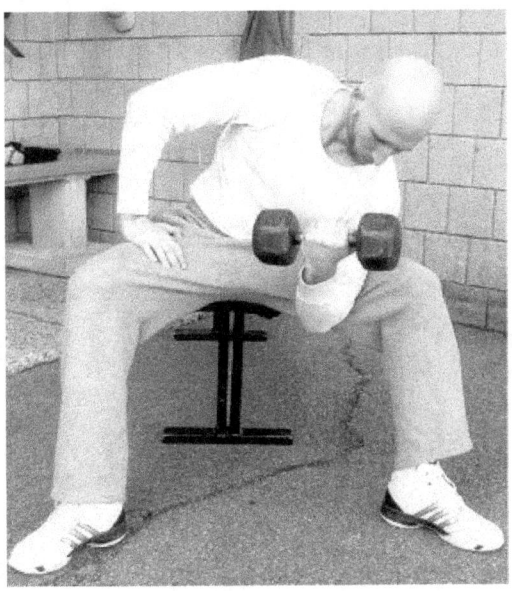

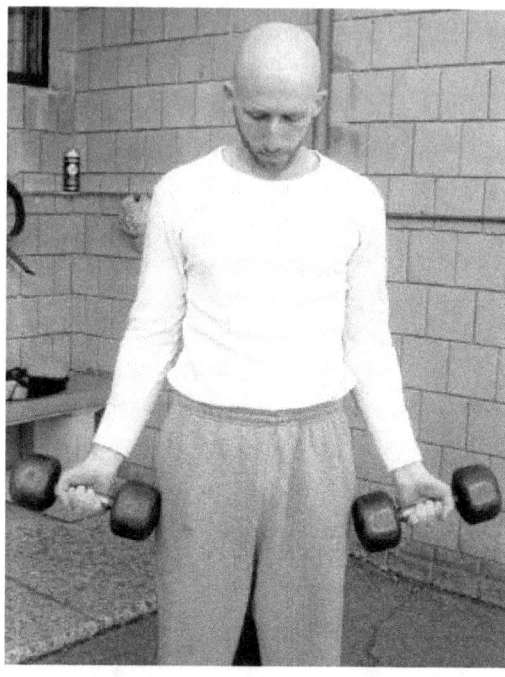

Curls -
(Targets the biceps) Stand tall with dumbells in each hand and palms out. Curl the weights upward simultaneously, pausing at the peak of contraction as you lower your arms back to the starting position.

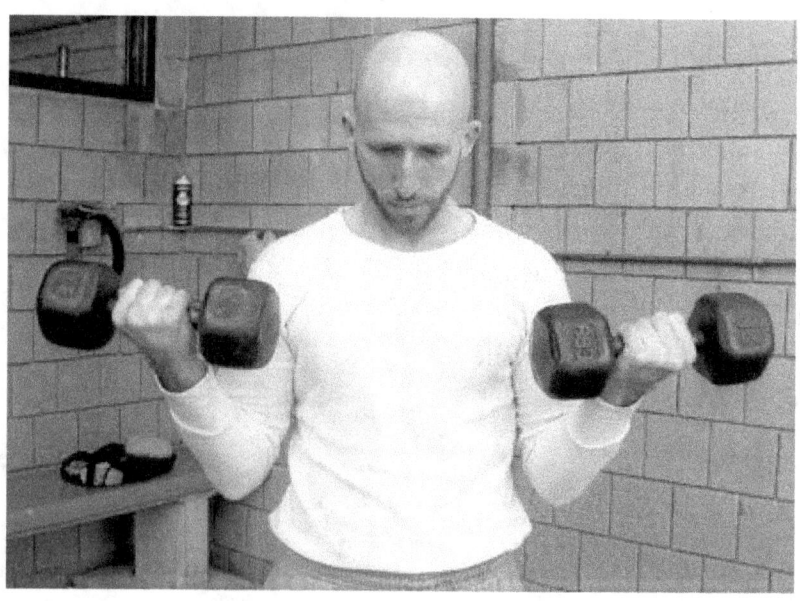

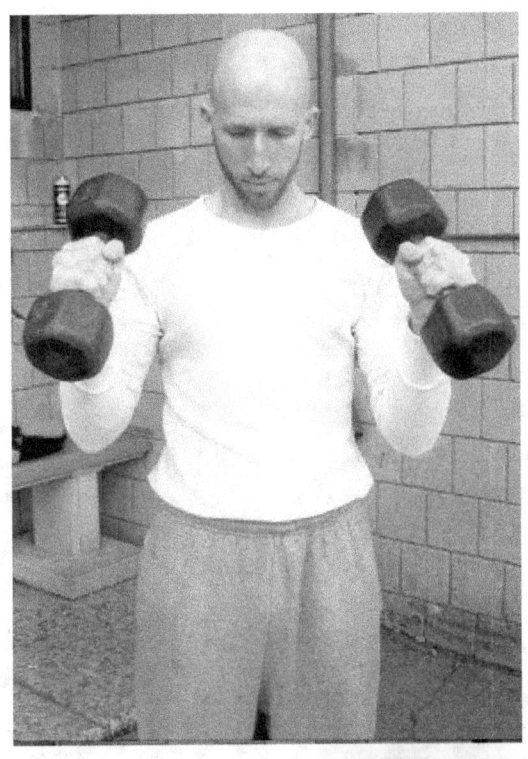

Hammer Curls-
(Targets the biceps) Stand tall with dumbells in each hand with your palms facing your sides. Curl the weights upward simultaneously. Pause at the peak of contraction and take three to five seconds to lower the weights on each rep.

Side Curls –
(Targets the biceps) Stand tall with dumbells in each hand. Allow your palms to face you. Curl the weights upward, almost bringing them together, pause, and slowly lower the weights to the starting position.

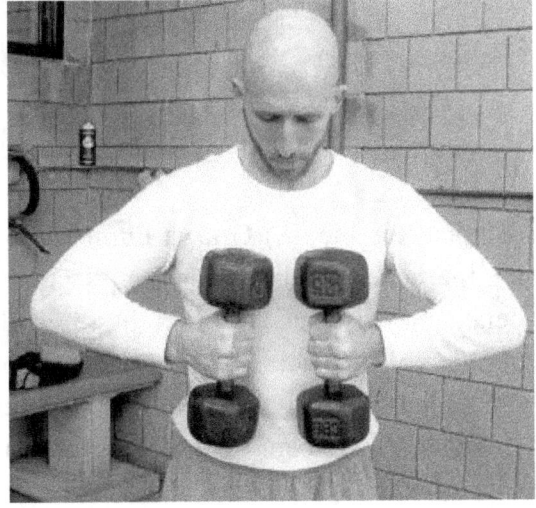

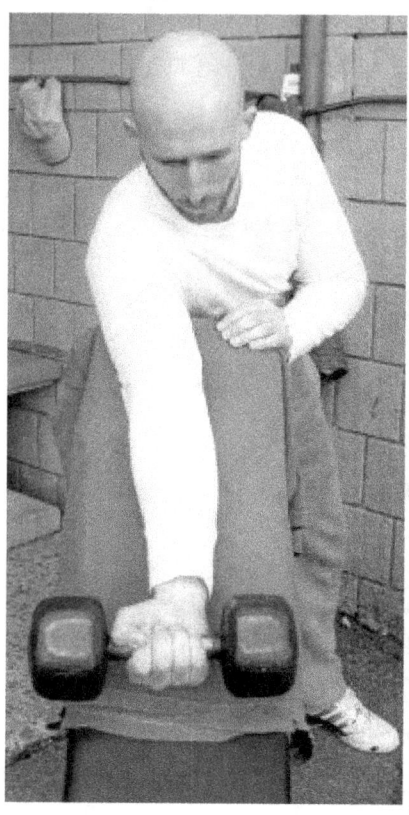 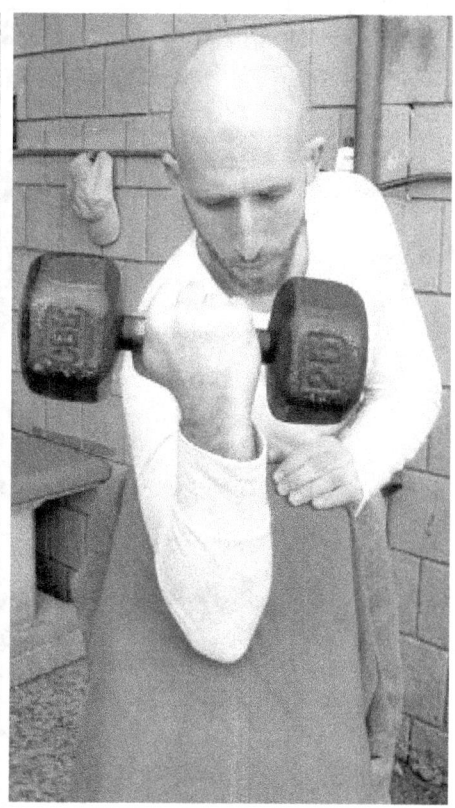

Concentration Curl –

(Targets the biceps) Grab a dumbell and place your arm on the incline bench so that your armpit almost touches the top of the bench. Slowly curl the weight upward. Pause at the peak of contraction and take five seconds to lower the weight on each rep. Don't lock out completely in between reps to ensure constant tension on the bicep. Repeat the same amount of reps on opposite side.

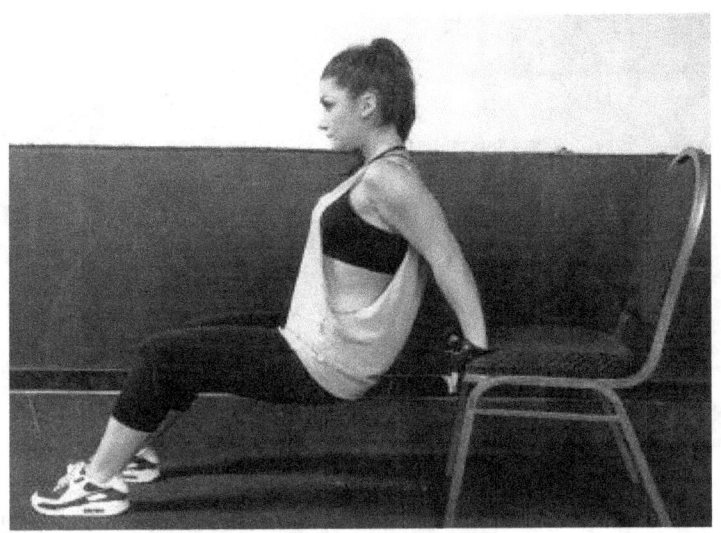

Seated Dips - (Targets the triceps) Place your palms on the bench or a chair, face away from the platform and extend your legs in front of you. Lower your body until your upper arms are parallel to the floor, but no lower. Extend your elbows to come up and return to the starting position.

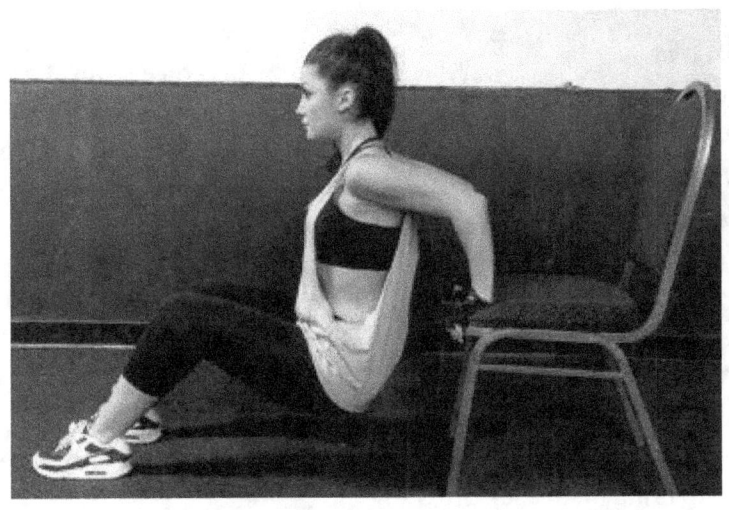

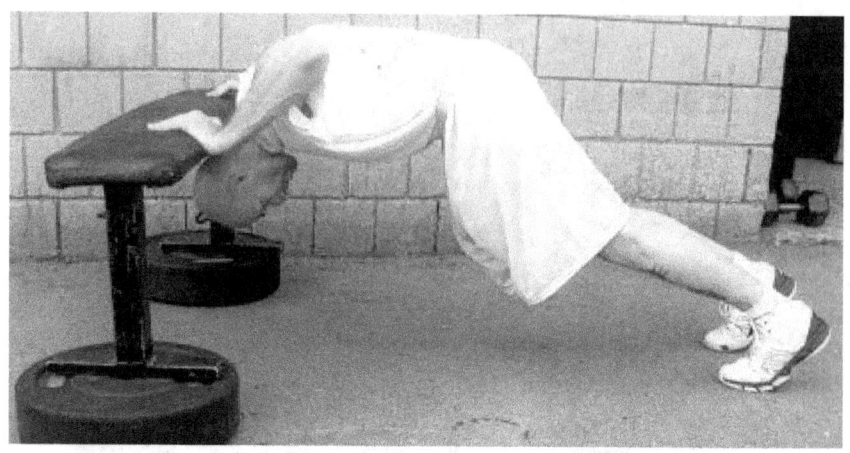

Tricep Extension-

(Targets the triceps) Use an elevated surface that's about waist high and can support your weight, such as a couch or a windowsill. Place your hands evenly over its edge, at shoulder width. Bend your elbows to lower your head beneath the object until you feel a stretch on your triceps, and then press yourself back to the starting position.

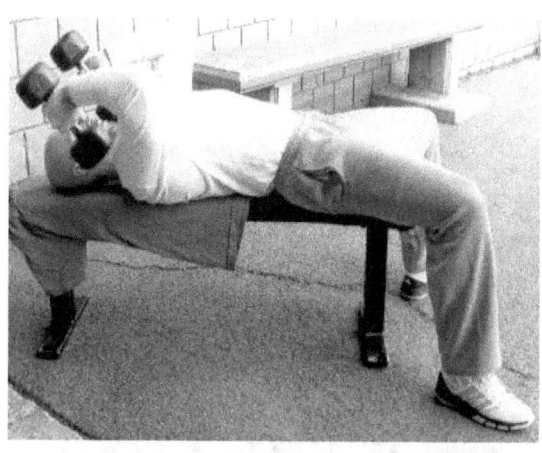

Lying Triceps Extension –

(Targets the triceps) Lie on a flat bench holding two dumbells. Fully extended your arms above you with your palms facing in, and your elbows over your chest. Keep your upper arms stationary and slowly lower the dumbells until they're close to your ears. Now, while keeping the elbows in and the upper arms stationary, use the triceps to bring them back up.

Lying Triceps Extension –

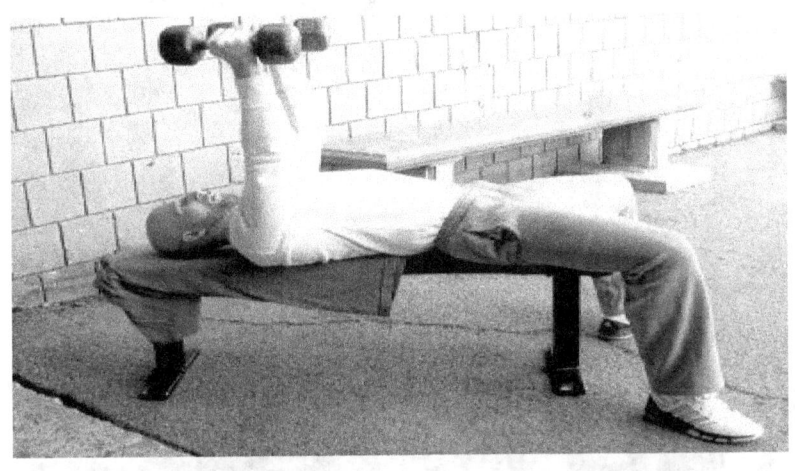

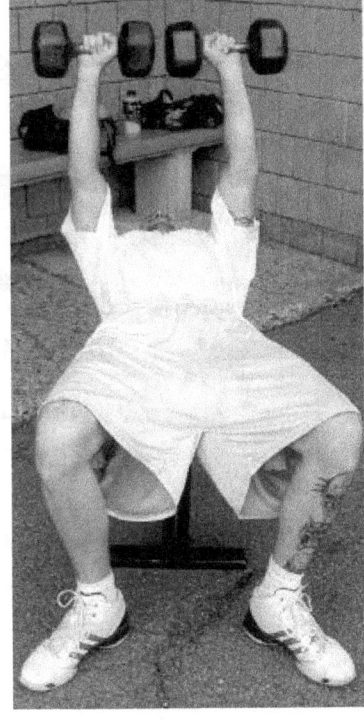

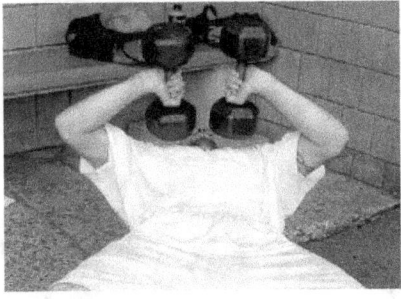

Tate Press-
(Targets the triceps) Lie on a flat bench holding two dumbells. With your arms fully extended above you, allow your palms to face your feet. Point your elbows outward and bend them to lower the weights almost to your chest. They should make an (L) shape. Once in the (L), extend your elbows to the starting position.

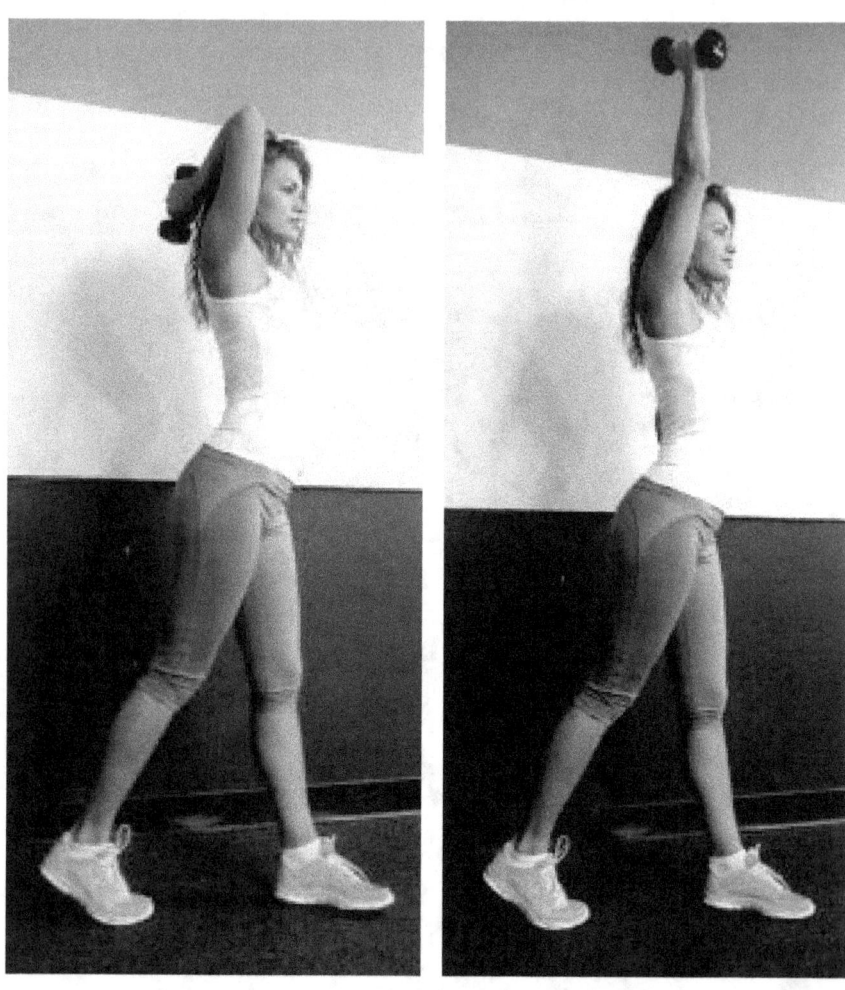

Overhead Extension –

(Targets the triceps) Grab a dumbell and raise your arm behind your head with your elbow bent. Extend your elbow straight over your head. Repeat the same amount of reps on opposite sides.

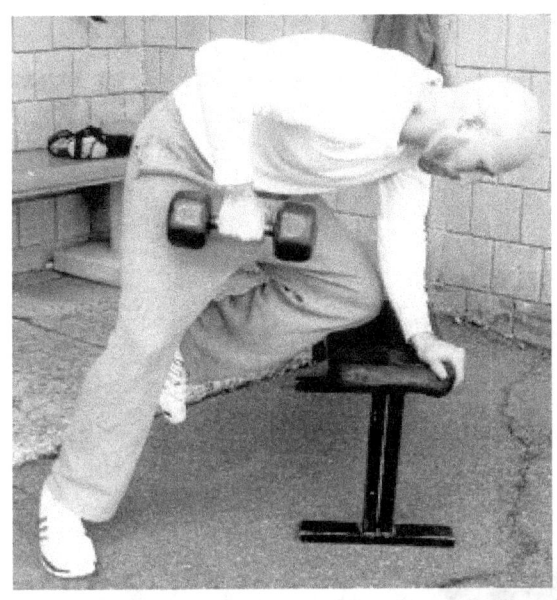

Kickbacks –
(Targets the triceps)
Grab a dumbell and lean forward until your back is almost parallel to the floor. With one leg positioned back and the front of your knee is on top of the bench or chair.

Place your elbow at your side and allow the rest of your arm with the dumbell in hand to hang down towards the floor. Draw your hand back until your triceps flex and slowly return to the starting position.

Repeat the same amount of reps on opposite sides.

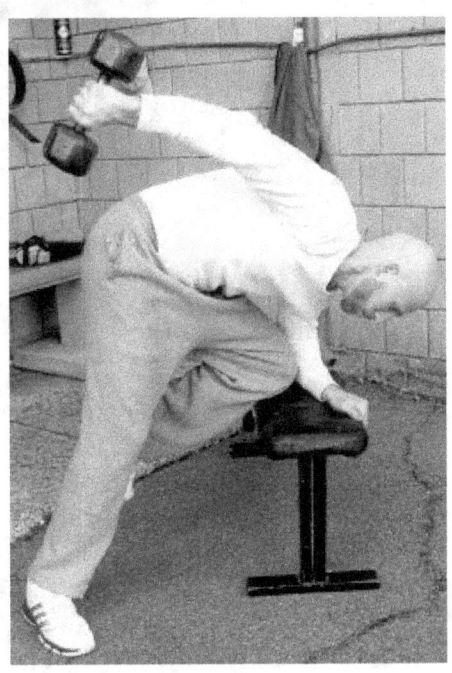

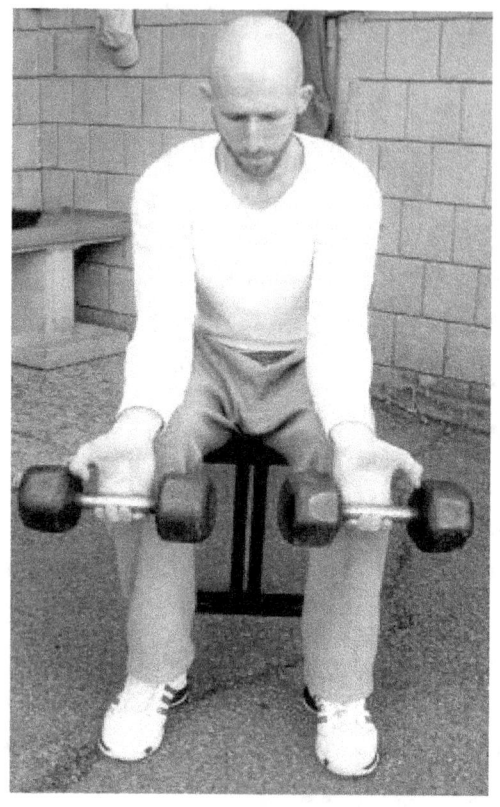

Wrist Curls –

(Targets the forearms) Hold a dumbell in each hand and sit on a bench. Rest your forearms on your thighs and allow your wrists to bend back over your knees allowing the weights to hang down.

Now, slightly open your hands and let the dumbells roll to your fingertips.

Then close your hands and curl the dumbells up by just flexing your wrists, then return to the starting position.

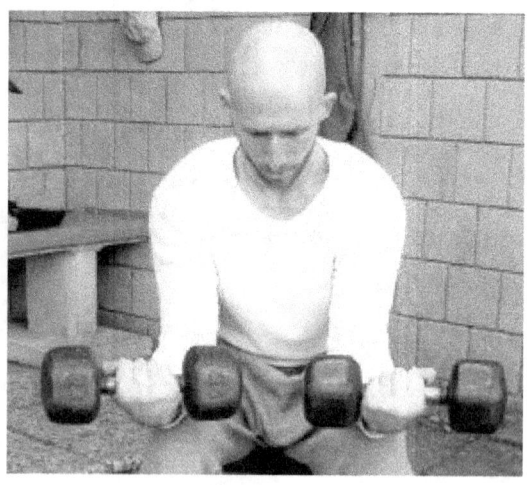

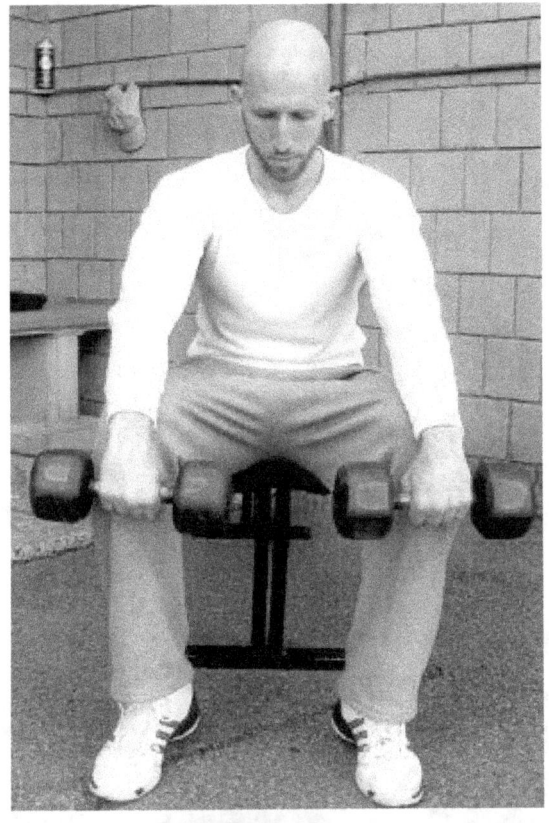

Reverse Wrist Curls-

(Targets the forearms) Hold a dumbell in each hand and sit on a bench.

Rest your forearms on your thighs with palms facing down and wrists over your knees.

Now extend your wrists to raise the back of your hands closer to your forearms, then return to the starting position.

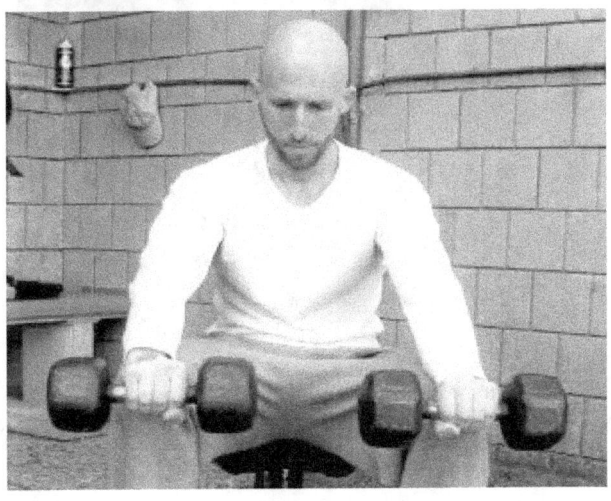

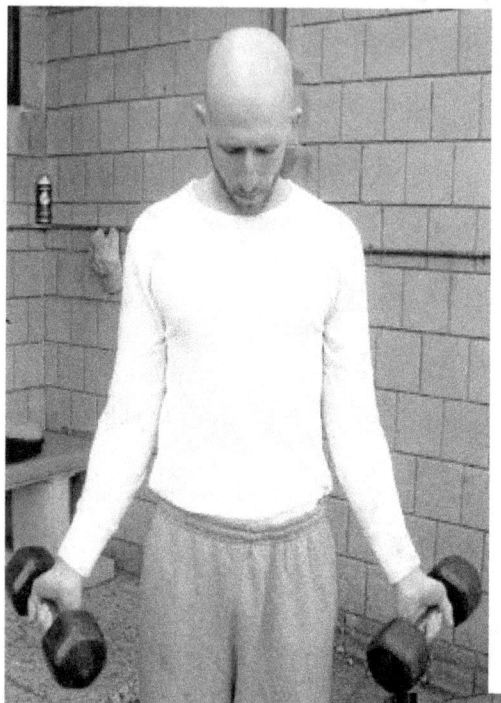

Forearm Twist-
(Targets the forearms) Stand tall with dumbells in each hand and palms out as far as possible. Rotate your forearms inward as far as you can.

Repeat this motion back and forth until failure.

Chest

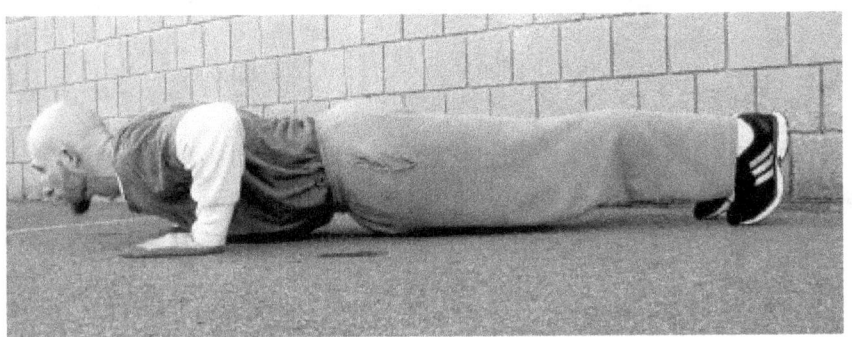

Standard Push-Up -
Lie on the floor with your hands apart and below your shoulders, feet together. Push your body up off the floor until your arms are extended. Keep your body rigid throughout the moves and don't let it sag. A perfect push-up is when you bring your chest an inch away from the floor, pause for a second, and then return to the starting position.

Close grip push-ups target the inner pecs, hands four inches apart. Medium grip push-ups targets your middle region. Your hands are shoulder width apart. Wide grip push-up targets the outer pecs, place your hands as wide apart as comfortable as possible.

Push-ups can also be performed with weights on your upper back. In order to squeeze the most out of every push-up, clench your glutes. This puts your pelvis in a neutral position, and stabilizes your spine and aligning your torso. It also ensures the efficient transfer of energy from your upper body to your lower body, which blasts your core and rear. In short, clenched butt cheeks are the link that holds the exercise together.

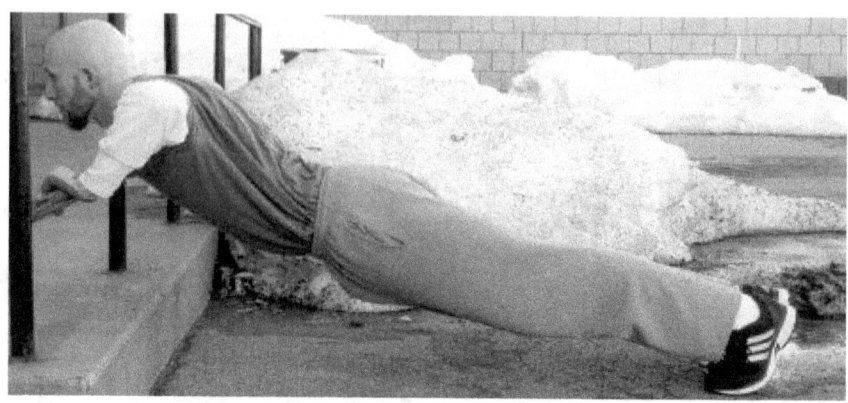

Incline Push-Up-

This particular exercise is a bit easier than a standard push-up. It's also a great method to work your way up instead of doing push-ups with your knees on the floor. Place your hands on a bench or any stable elevated surface. Prop yourself up on the balls of your feet and slowly lower your body as far as possible, pause for a second and return to the starting position.

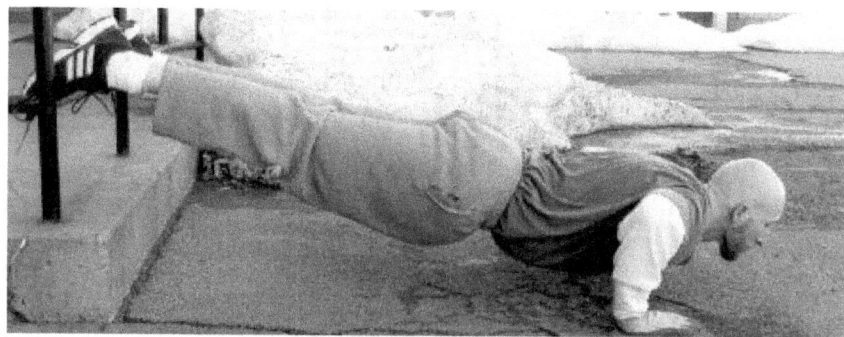

Decline Push-Up – This particular exercise is a bit harder than a standard push-up. Place your feet on a bench or any stable elevated surface (the higher you go, the harder it gets). With your hands on the floor wider than shoulder width. Keep your head neutral and your abs tight. Lower your body until your chest almost touches the floor, pause for a second and return to the starting position.

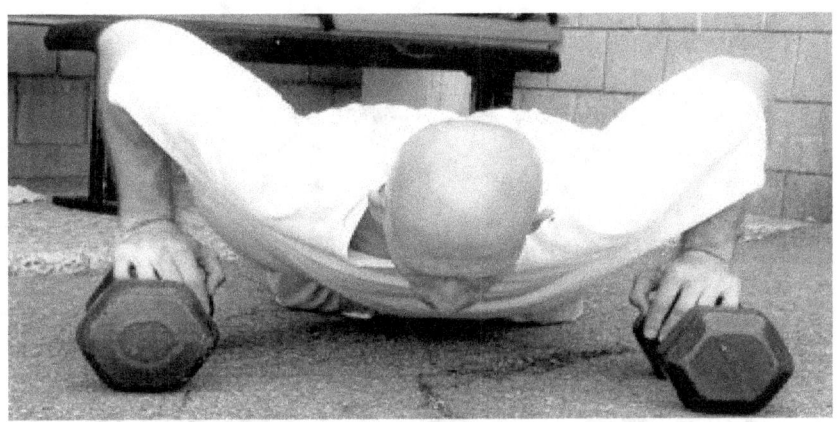

Deep Push-Up – Even though you're going a little lower and deeper with this move than you would with a standard push-up, keep your back straight and your abs tight at all times. Going deeper, you'll activate more muscle fibers, thereby improving growth potential. Place your hands on two dumbells, or full boxes. Bend your elbows and slowly lower your chest toward the floor between the dumbells until it is fully stretched. Pause for a second and return to the starting position.

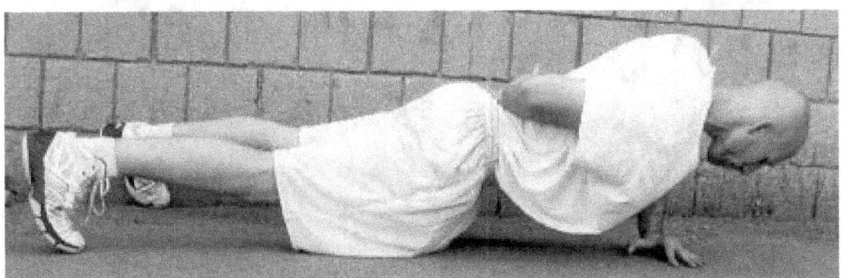

One Arm Push-Up - Get into a standard push-up position, only spread your feet a bit wider than shoulder width apart. Take one hand and place it behind your back, while spreading the fingers of your working hand wide apart for balance. Tuck your elbow into your rib cage. Slowly lower your body as far as you can go and press forcefully back to the starting position. Repeat the same amount of reps on the opposite side.

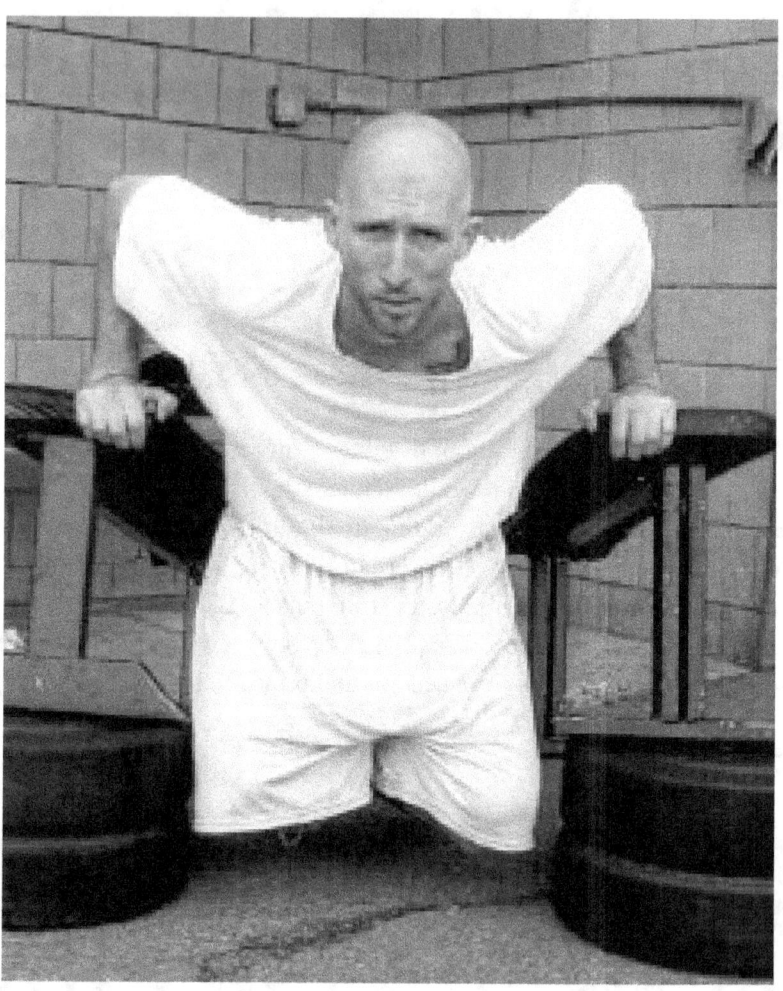

Dips-

Find two stable, equally high surfaces. This may be something like a pair of parallel bars or two chairs. Place your palms on each surface and straighten your arm. Cross your ankles and bend your knees until your lower legs are parallel to the floor. Bend your elbows and slowly lower your body as far as possible. With your knees suspended in the air above the floor, push yourself back up into the starting position.

Dumbell Bench Press –

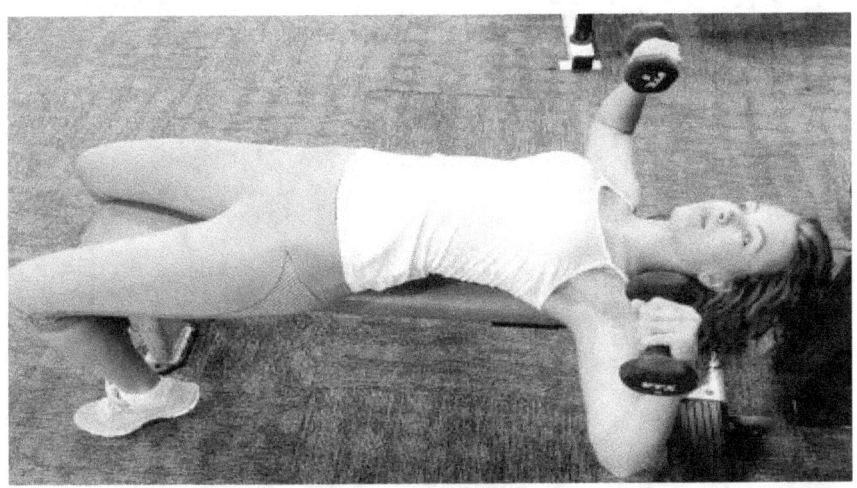

Lie flat on the bench, feet on the floor. Grab a dumbell in each hand and hold the weights at shoulder level. Press the dumbells straight over your chest, turning your hands inward during the motion.

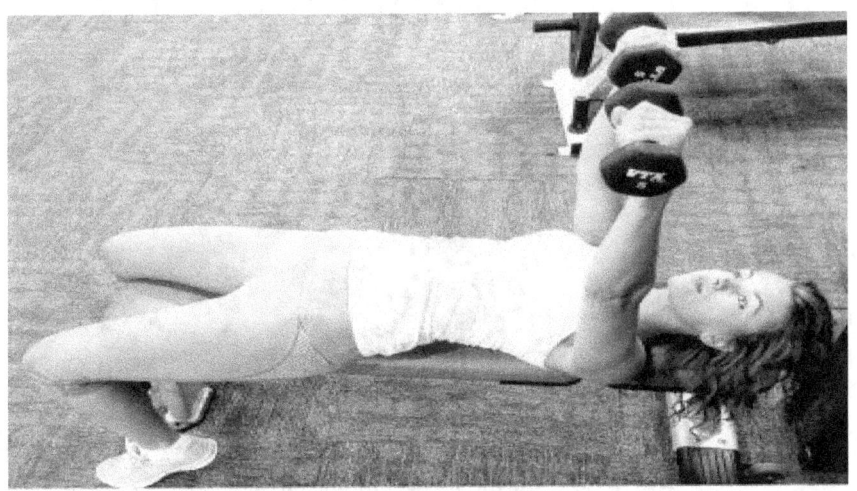

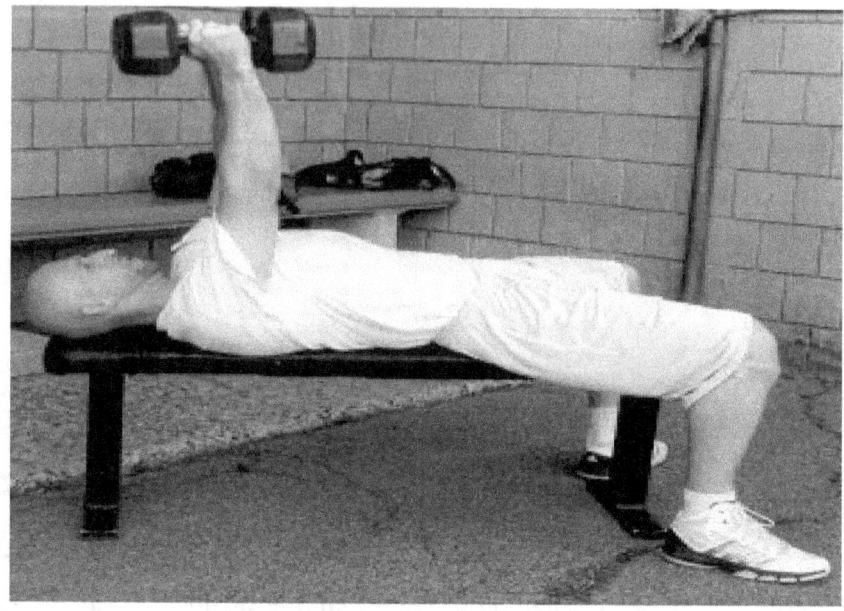

Fly's -

Lie flat on the bench, with your feet on the floor. With a dumbell in each hand, your arms should be lightly bent straight up for the start position. Make sure your palms are facing each other. Keeping a slight bend in your arms, slowly move dumbells away from each other, allowing your arms to lower, but they will

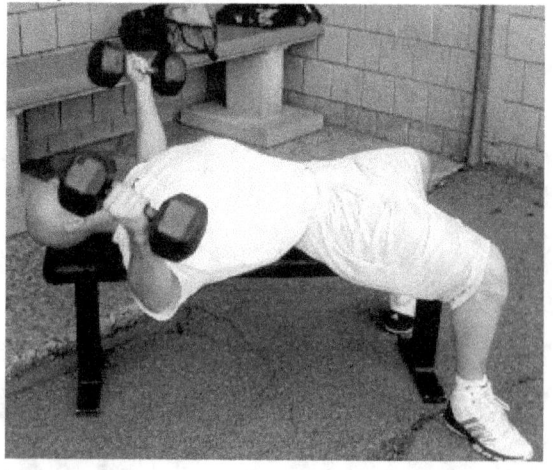

remain slightly bent. Lower your arms until a comfortable stretch is felt in the chest. Raise your arms back up along the same path to the starting position as if you are hugging a tree.

94

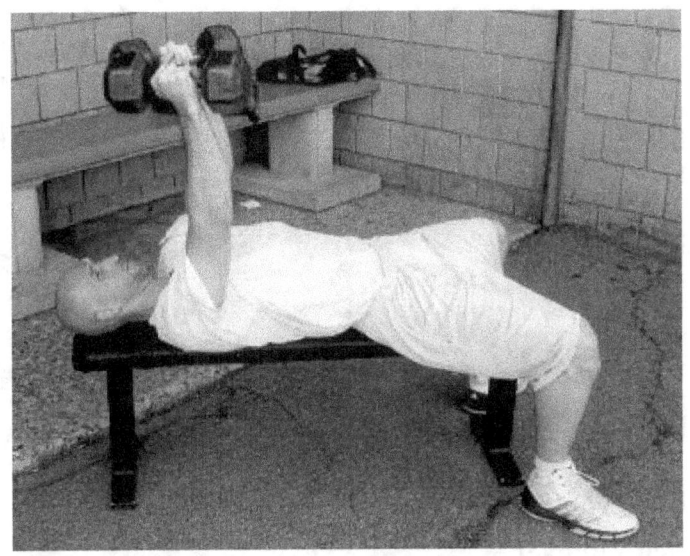

Champagnes-

Lie flat on the bench, with your feet on the floor and a dumbell in each hand. Hold the weights at arms-length above your chest with your palms facing each other and dumbells connected. Slowly lower the dumbells bringing them within an inch from your chest, once parallel, raise the weights back up to the starting position.

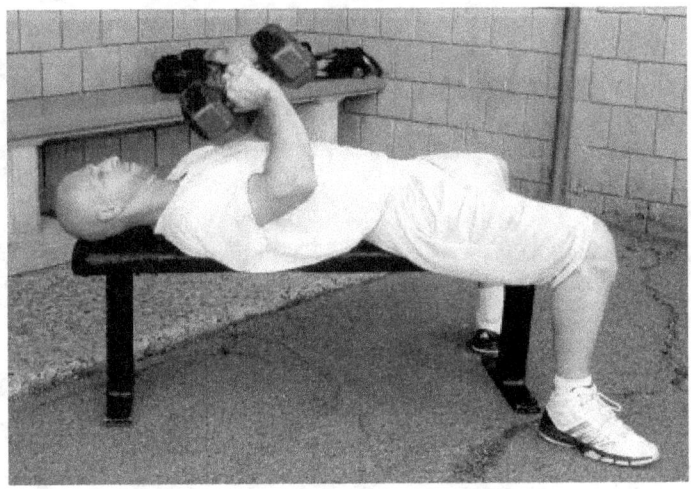

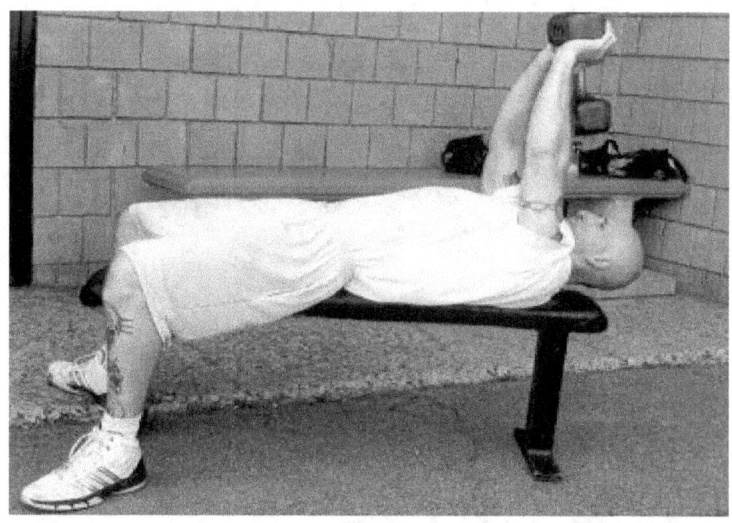

Dumbell Pullover –

Lie flat on the bench with your head at the very end. Hold a dumbell at arms-length above your head with hands flat against the inside plate. Keeping your elbows in a locked position, lower the weight in a semicircular motion behind your head, going as low as possible. Once you can't go any lower, raise the weight back up over your head, still keeping elbows locked. Return to the starting position.

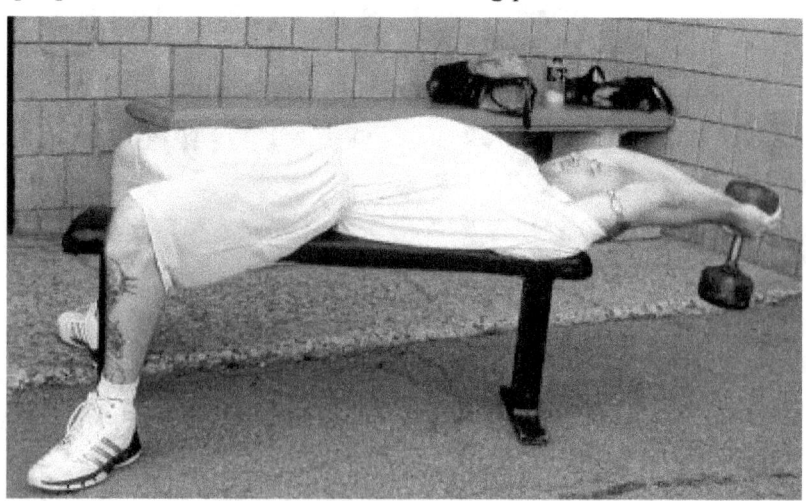

Shoulders

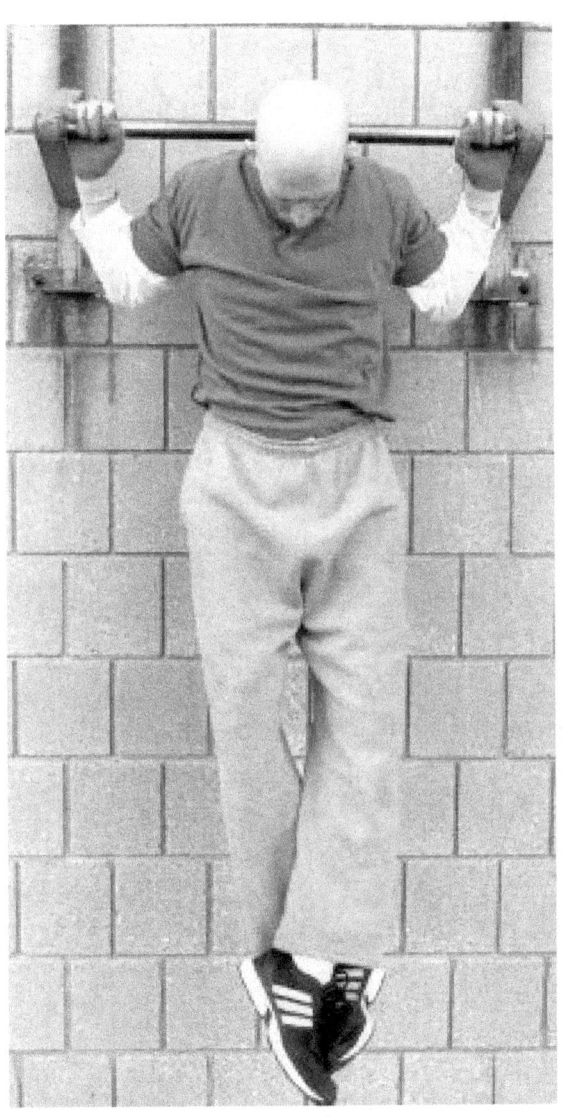

Behind the neck Pull Up –

With your hands wider than shoulder width apart, grab the pull-up bars width with your palms facing out. Rest your chin on your chest and cross your ankles.

Bend your elbows and pull your body straight up so that the back of your head goes over the bar.

Pause for a second and return to the starting position.

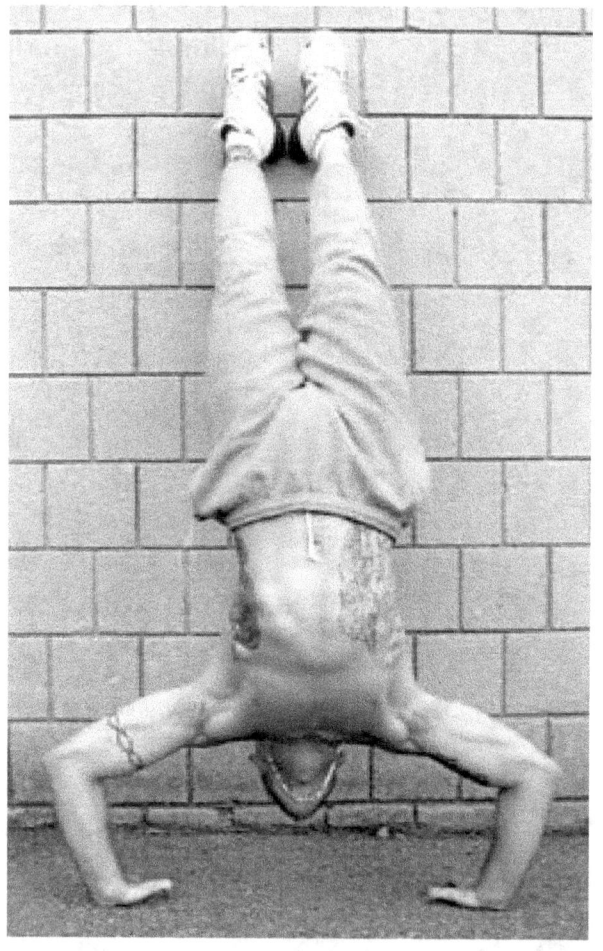

Hand Stand Push-Up –
Squat down, facing a sturdy wall and place your hands on the floor about ten inches away from the wall. Lean forward and put your head on the floor.

(You can use a small pillow for a cushion). Kick off with your leg and bring both legs on the wall, keep your body in a perfectly straight line from your hands to your feet. In a slow and controlled motion push with your arms and bring yourself up until your elbows are nearly locked. Slowly lower yourself until your head almost touches the floor.

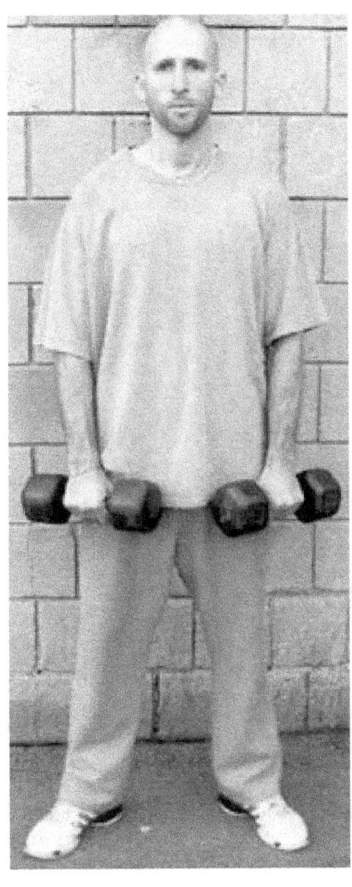 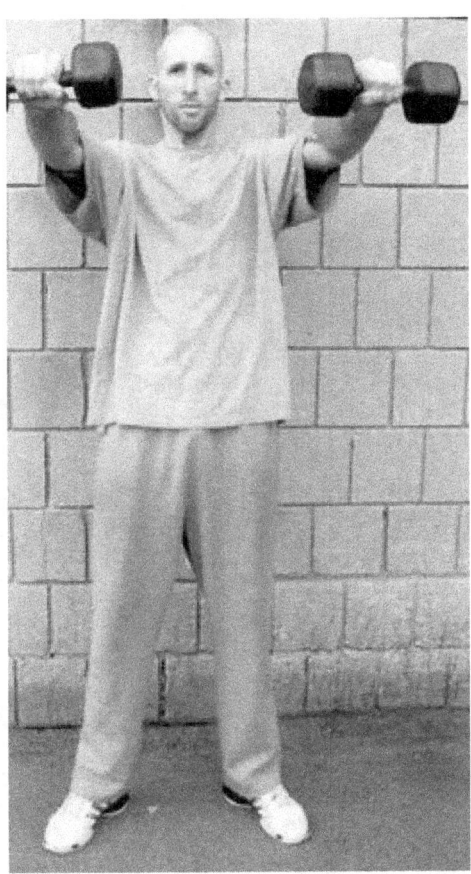

Front Lateral Raise –

Grab two dumbells and stand with your feet shoulder width apart. Rest your arms at your sides with your palms facing inwards. Raise both arms straight out to your sides, until they are at shoulder level. Pause for a second and slowly lower your hands back down to your sides. (You may also work one arm at a time for higher reps).

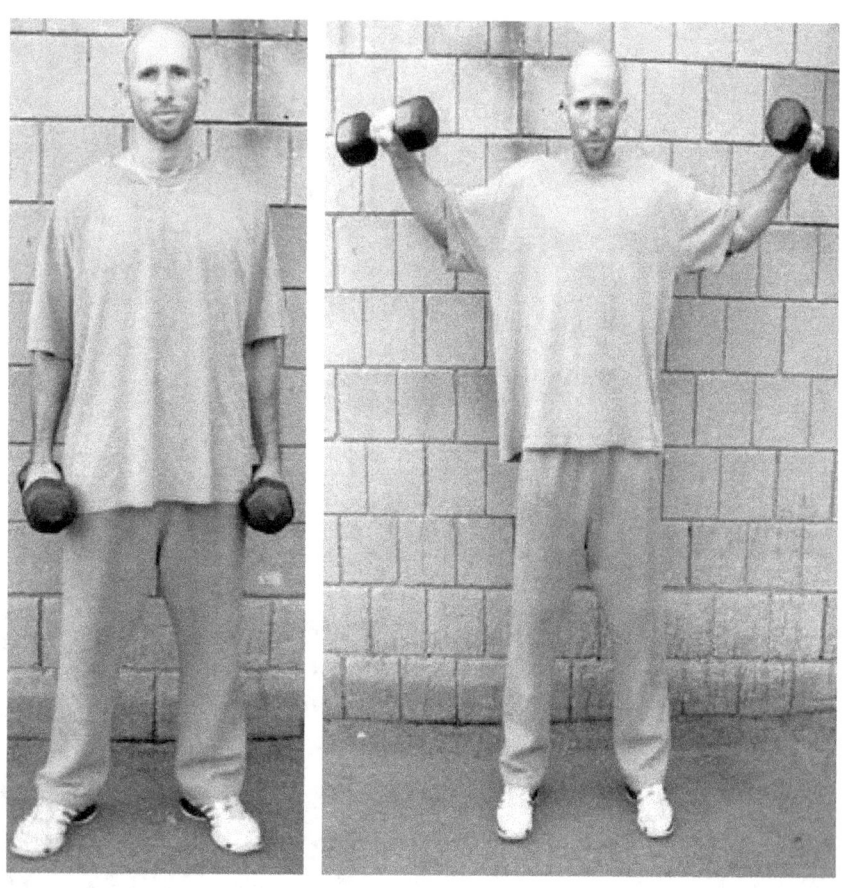

Side Lateral Raise -
Grab two dumbells and stand with your feet shoulder width apart. Place your arms at your sides with your palms facing inwards. Raise both arms straight out in front of you until they are at shoulder level. Pause for a second and slowly lower your hands back down to your sides. (You may also work one arm at a time for higher reps).

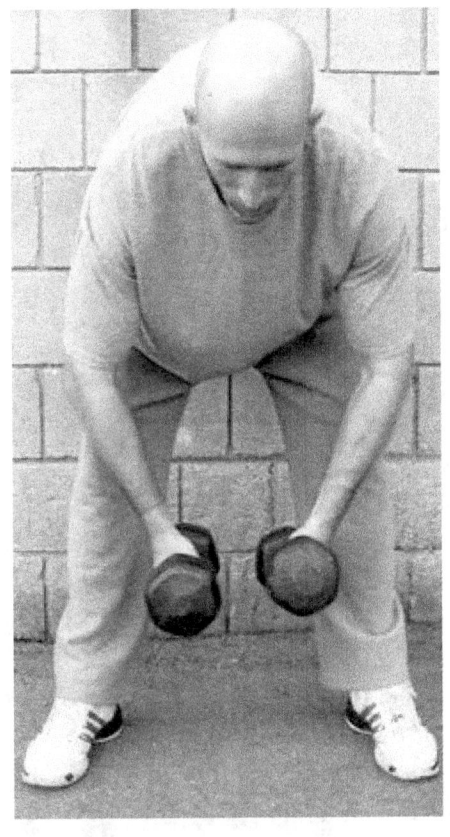

Back Lateral Raise -
Grab two dumbells and stand with your feet shoulder width apart. With your arms in front of you, turn your palms facing inward. Keep your back, arms and knees slightly bent and lean forward until your back is almost parallel with the floor.

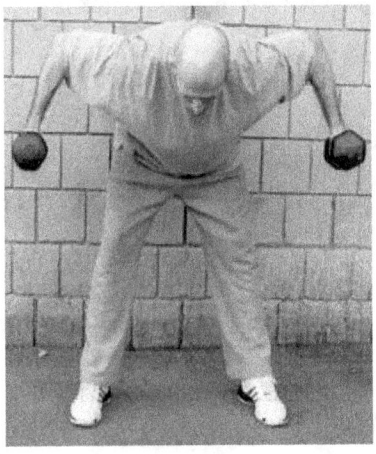

Raise both arms out to your sides as far as you can. Pause for a second and slowly lower your hands back down.

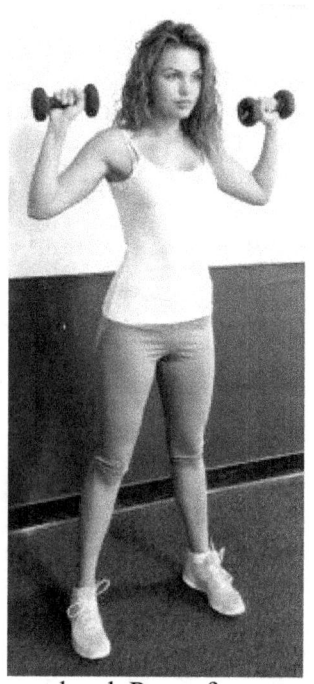

Overhead Dumbell Press-

Grab two dumbells and sit on the incline bench with your back flat against it. Raise the weights equal with your shoulders. Make sure your triceps become parallel with the floor and your palms are facing out. Press the dumbells straight

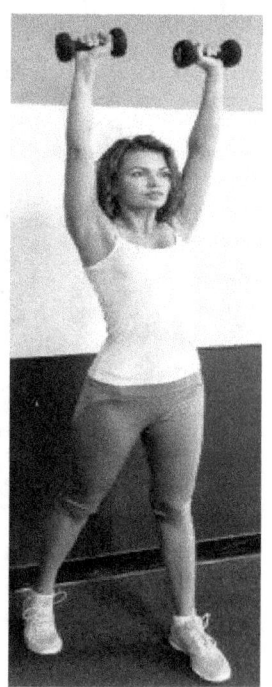

overhead. Pause for a second and slowly lower the weights back down.

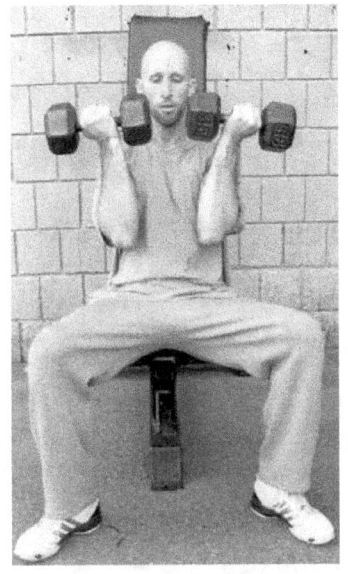 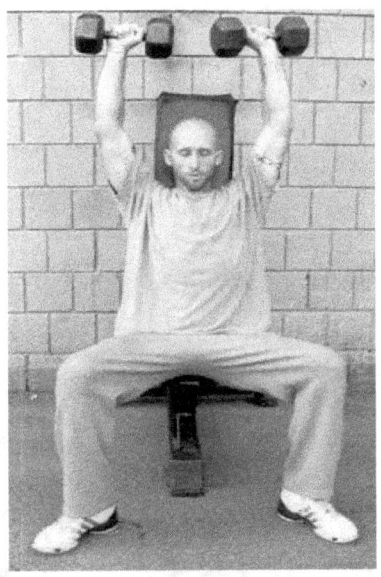

Rotating Dumbell Press –

Grab two dumbells and sit on the incline bench with your back flat against it. Bring the weights at shoulder level so your triceps become parallel with the floor. With your palms facing you begin to press the weights overhead and rotate your palms to face forward as you go up. Pause for a second and slowly lower the weights back down.

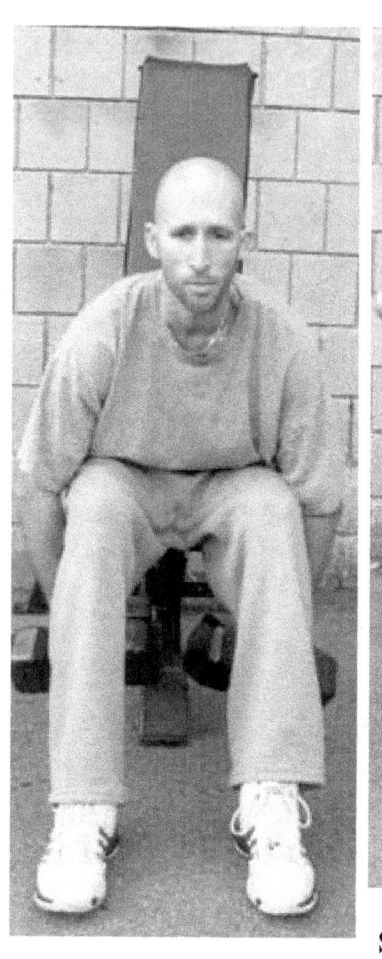 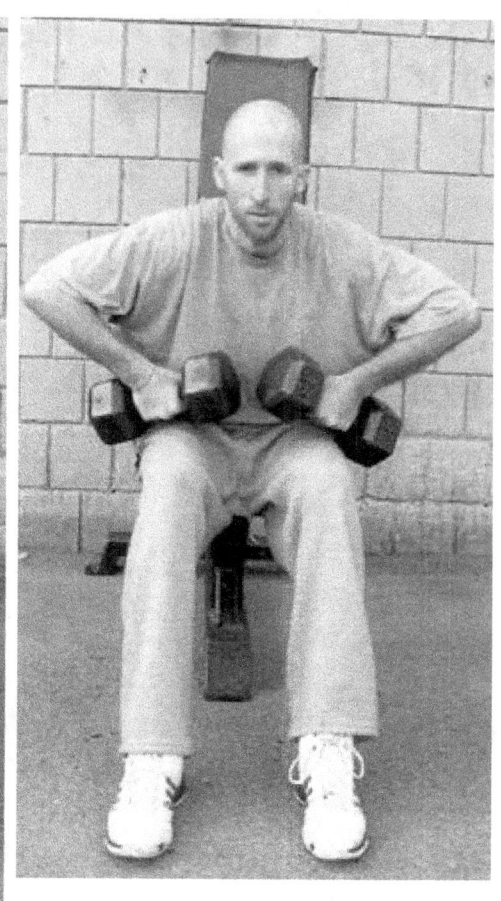

Seated Dumbell Curves –

Hold a dumbell in each hand, with your palms facing inwards. Sit on the edge of a bench, and keep your lower back flat. Lean forward and bring both dumbells together over your thighs in a circular motion. Pause for a second and return to the starting position.

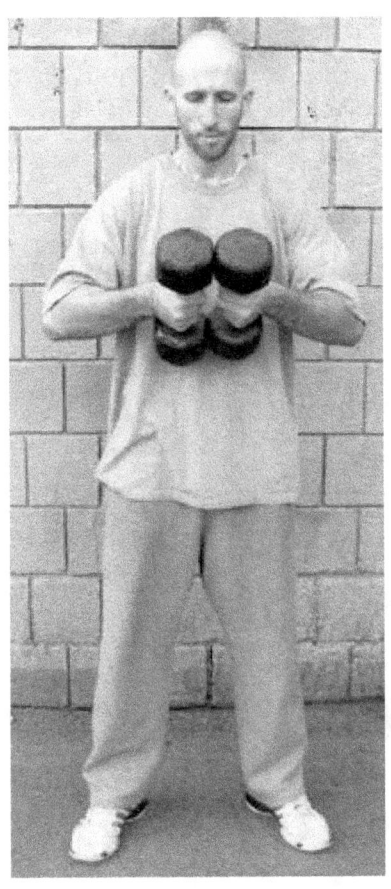 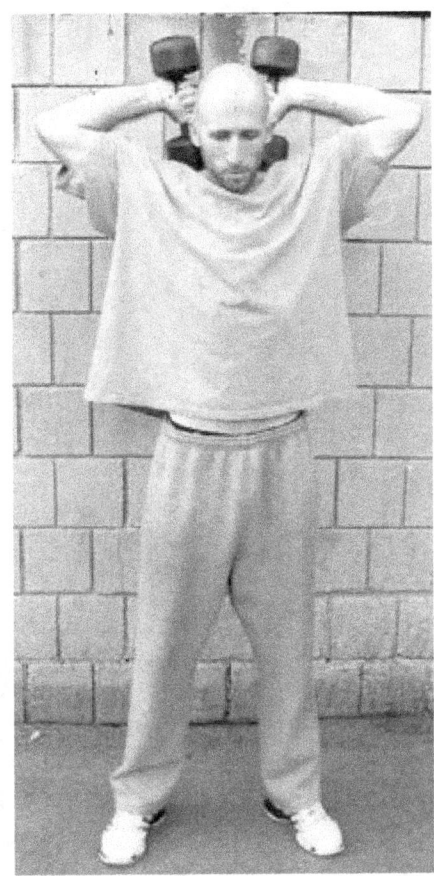

Butterfly Dumbell Twists –

Grab two dumbells and stand with your feet shoulder width apart. Bend your elbows and curl the weights to your chest with your palms facing each other. From this position bring the dumbells behind your neck in a circular motion while rotating your palms to face forward. Pause for a second and return to the starting position.

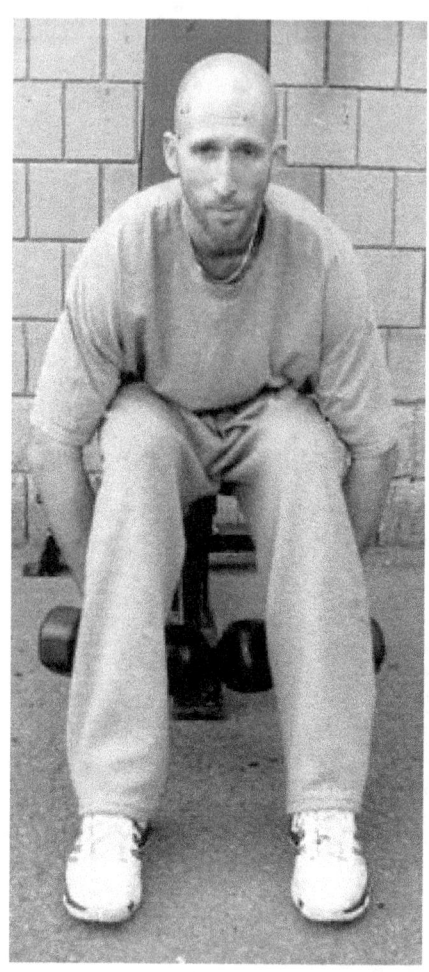 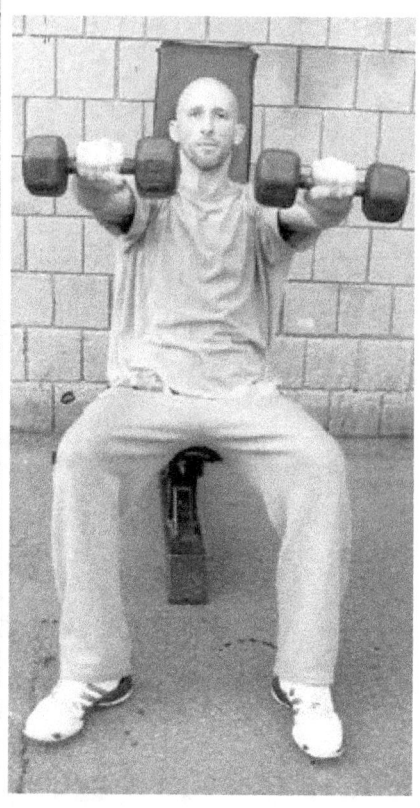

Seated Dumbell Clean -

Sit on the edge of the bench, holding a dumbell in each hand with your palms facing inwards. Keeping your lower back flat, lean forward. Explosively straighten your body and raise your arms, bringing the weights at shoulder level and your triceps parallel to the floor. Pause for a second and return to the starting position.

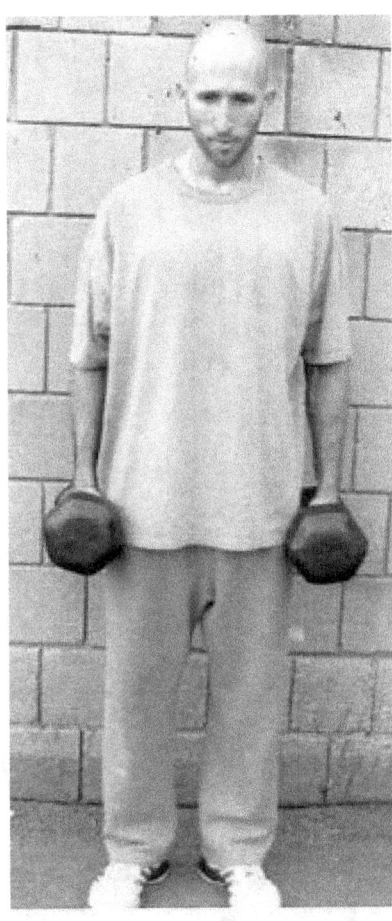 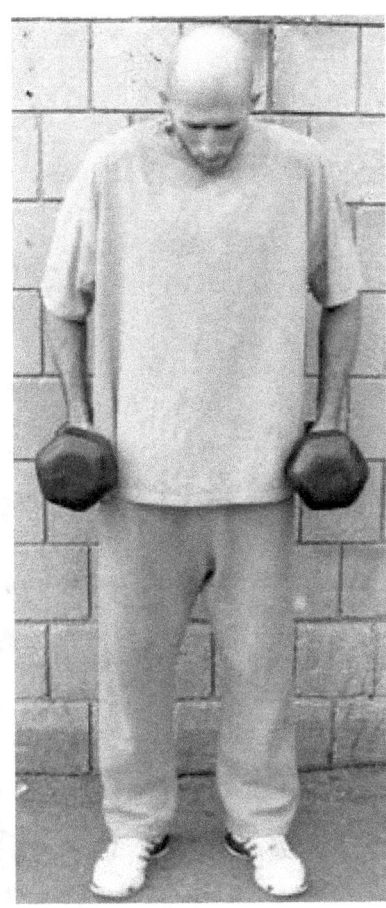

Dumbell Shrugs-

Stand with your feet hip width apart. Holding a dumbell in each hand, allow your palms to face your sides. Raise your shoulders as if you are trying to connect them to your ears. Pause for two seconds and return to the starting position.

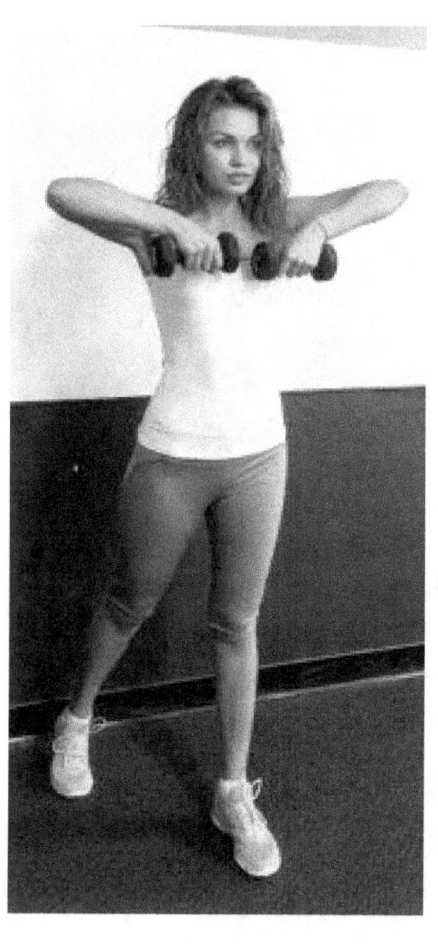
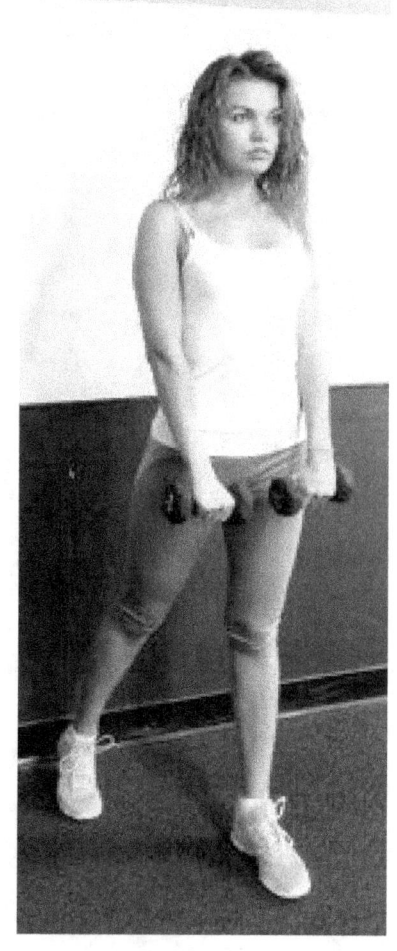

Dumbell High Pull-

Grab two dumbells and stand with your feet shoulder width apart. Place your arms in front of your thighs with your palms facing backwards. Raise the weights to your shoulders with elbows wide apart. Pause for a second and return to the starting position.

BACK

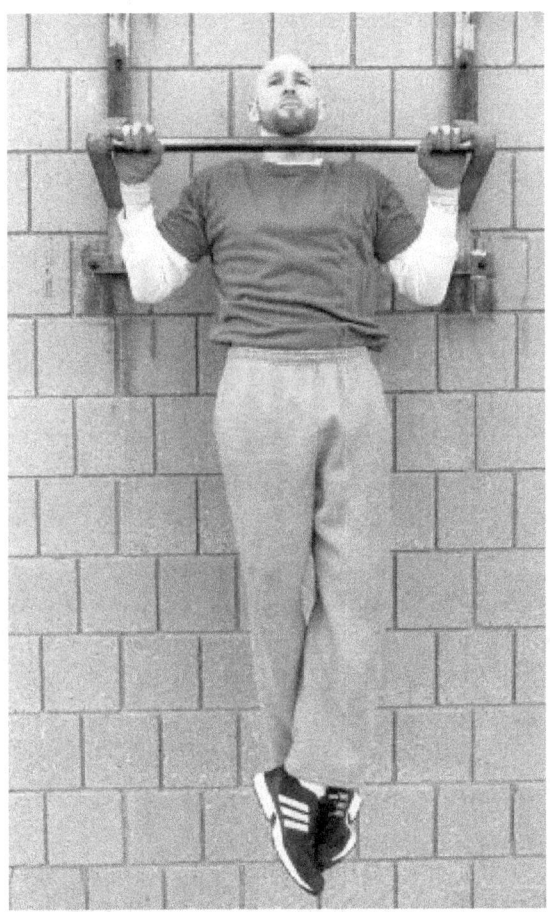

Wide Grip Pull-up –

Grab the pull-up bar wider than shoulder width. With your palms facing outward, cross your ankles. Bend your elbows and pull your body straight up, bringing your chin over the bar. Pause for a second and return to the starting position.

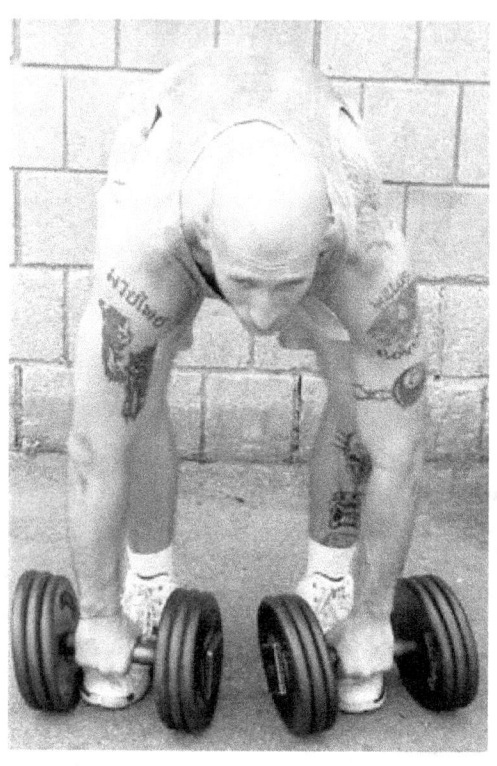 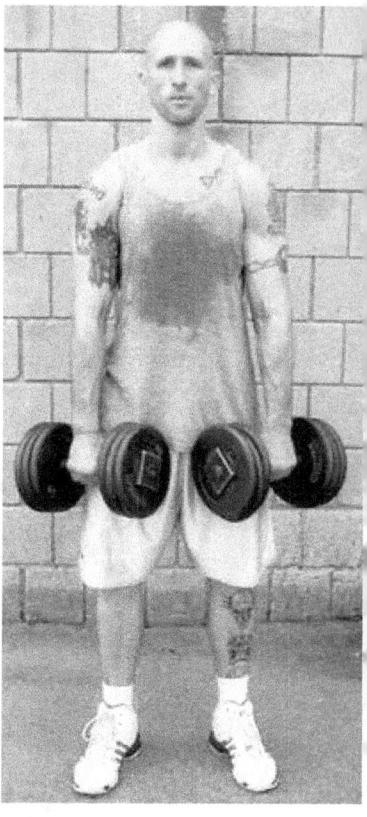

Dumbell Dead Lift-

Grab two dumbells and stand with your feet shoulder width apart
Place your arms by your sides with your palms facing inward.
Your back and knees should be straight and shoulders pulled
back. Bend forward at the hips, slowly lowering the weights
down. Pause for two seconds and return to the starting position.

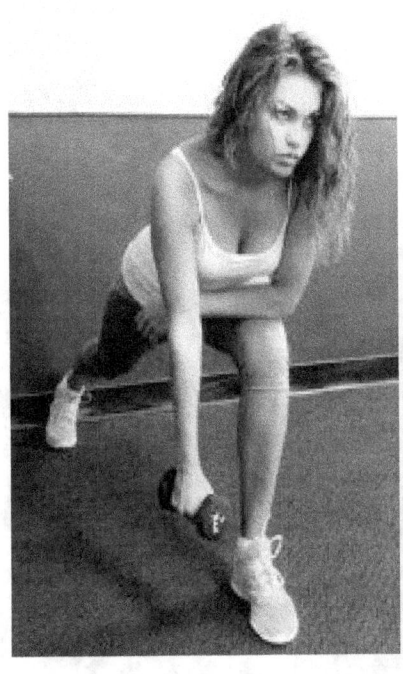 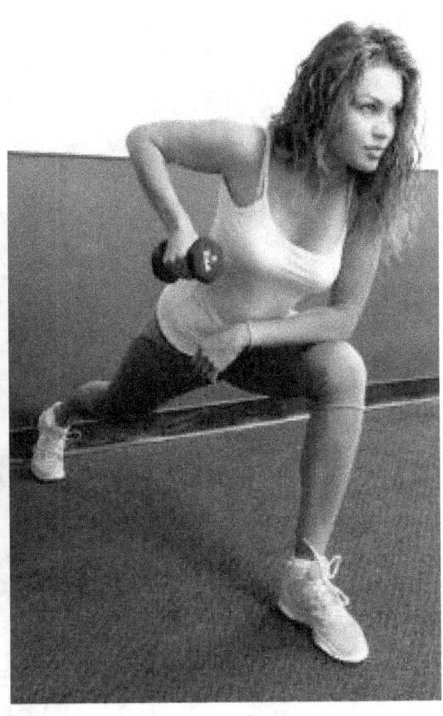

One Arm Row -

Hold a dumbell in your right hand and stand with your feet shoulder width apart. With your left foot in front of you. Bend your hips back until your torso is parallel to the floor and your working arm hanging down with your thumb pointing forward. Draw your shoulder blade back and roll the weight to your side.

Pause for a second and return to the starting position.
Repeat the same amount of reps on the opposite side.

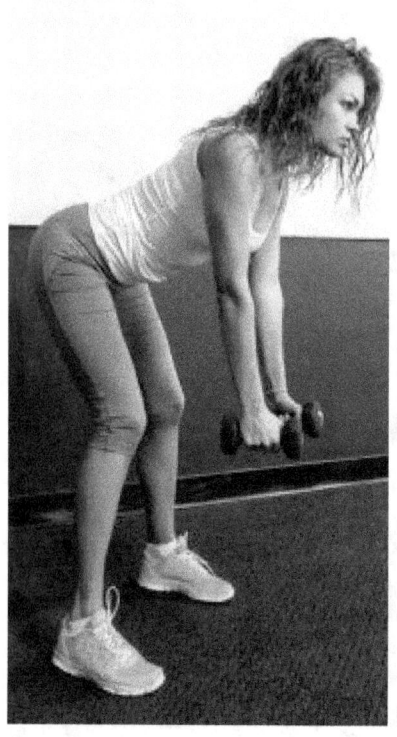
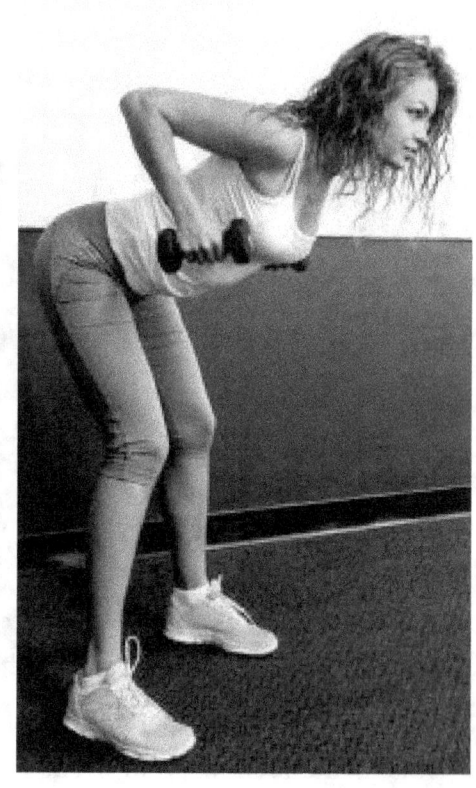

Bent Over Row-

Grab two dumbells and stand with your feet shoulder width apart. With your arms in front of your thighs allow your palms to face backwards. Bend your hips back until your torso is parallel to the floor. Draw your shoulder blades back and roll the weights to your chest.

Pause for a second and return to the starting position.

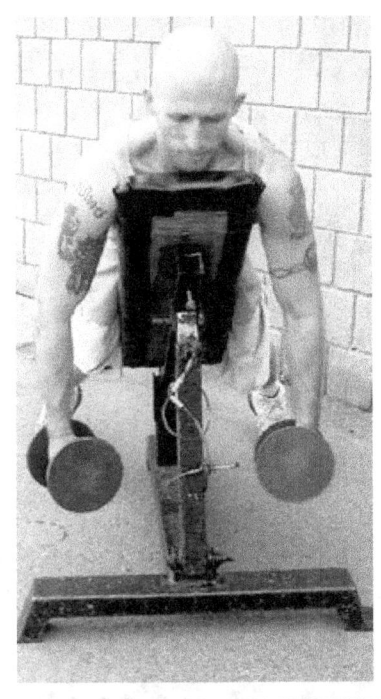

Lying Lateral Raise-

Lie down on the incline bench, with your chest facing downward. With a dumbell in each hand, allow your palms to face each other. Bring your arms out to your sides so your palms face down in the top position.

Pause for a second and return to the starting position.

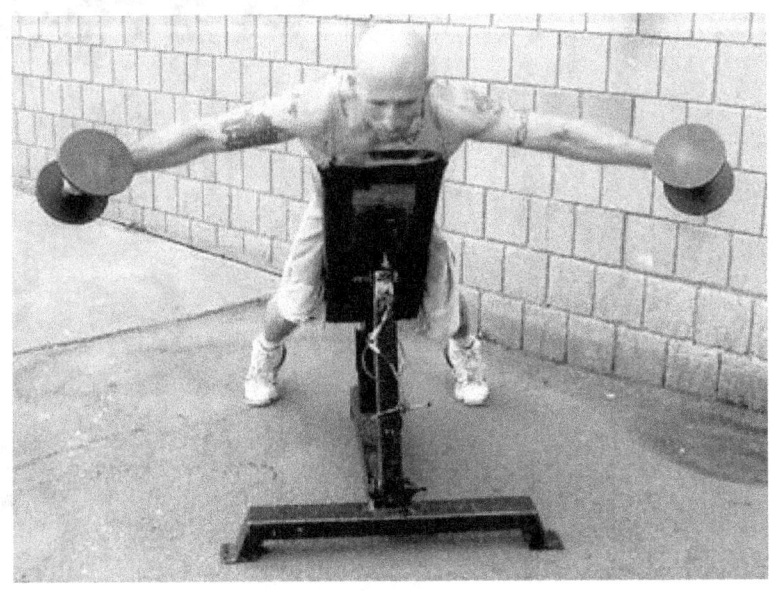

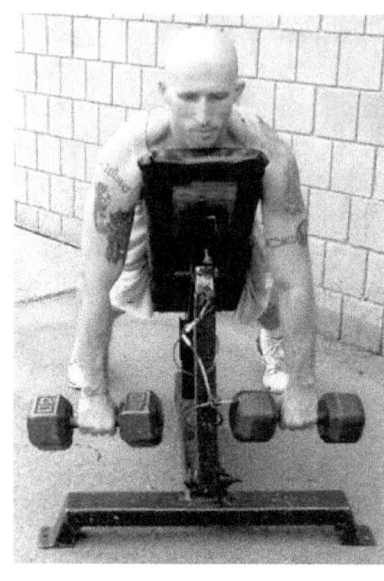

Incline Supported Row –

Lie down on the incline bench, with your chest down. With a dumbell in each hand allow your palms to face your feet. Squeeze your shoulder blades together and roll the weights to your sides.

Pause for a second and return to the starting position.

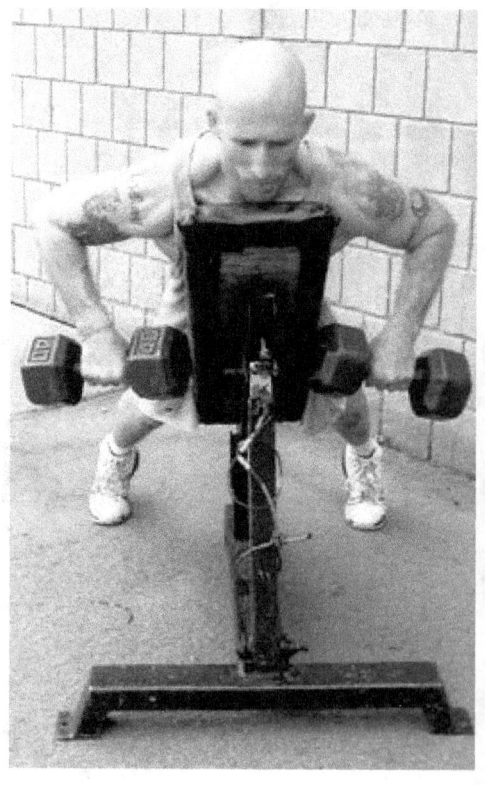

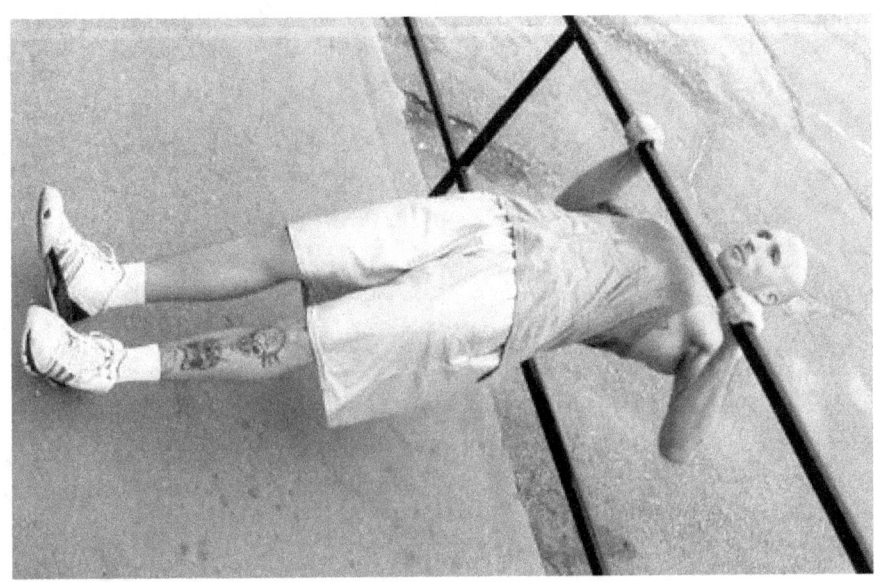

Inverted Row –

Lie on your back so that your chest is underneath the bench. Reach up and grip the side of the bench over handed. Keep your body in a straight line and pull yourself up toward the underside of the bench, so that only your heels stay on the floor.

Pause for two seconds and return to the starting position.

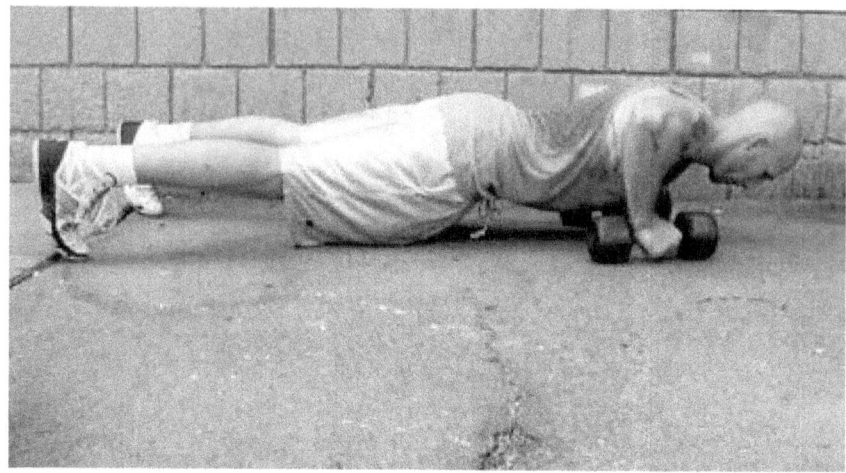

Dumbell Push-up Row -

Grab two dumbells and get into a push-up position. Keep your body as straight as a plank of wood from head to toe. Draw your shoulder blade back and roll the weight to your side with your right hand. Return to the starting position and perform a push-up.

Now roll the dumbell to your side with your left hand. Return to the starting position and perform a push-up.

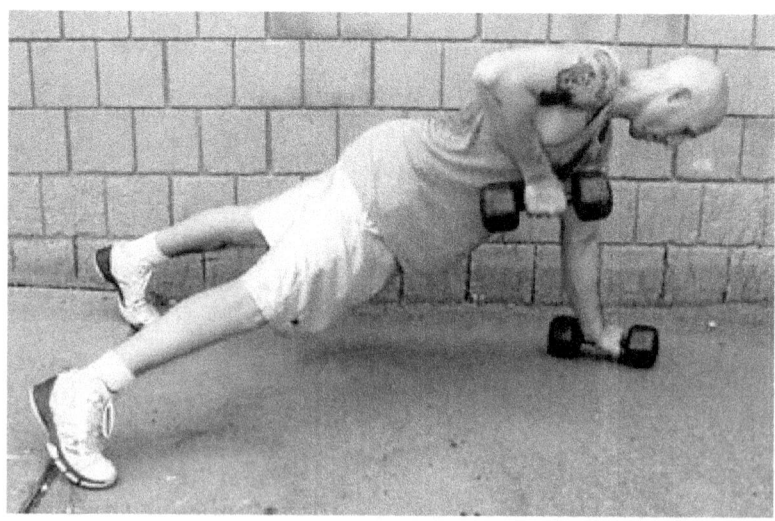

Nutritional Knowledge

People today consume way more food than they actually need. Everyone knows that. Our modern world conspires to make us fat and keep us fat. The food scientists combine sugar, salt and fat so that "enough" is never actually enough. And people end up stuffing themselves even when they don't feel hungry. As important as exercise is, it runs a distant second to the first change you need to make. That change would be to clean up your diet and lower your caloric intake. Proper nutrition is the main key to your long- term fitness goal. A good workout and crappy diet will not get you anywhere. To reach your set goals you need to develop a lifetime of healthy eating habits by applying dietary fundamentals that will help you reach them.

Always keep in mind that your diet is at least eighty percent of your success or failure. This chapter will teach you everything you need to know about healthy eating and balancing quality sources of protein, carbohydrates and fats. So before you go on to the next page, you can start by eliminating soda, candy and junk food out of your system.

DIGESTIVE SYSTEM

Food provides us with fuel to live, energy to work and play, and the raw materials to build new cells. All the different varieties of food we eat are broken down by our digestive system and transported to every part of our body by our circulatory system.

Digestive Tract- This long tube is the main part of the digestive system, it's roughly nine meters in length, all through the middle of the body. It starts at the mouth, where food and liquids enter the body, and ends at the annus, which is where leftover food and wastes exits the body. The succession of the digestive tract is as follows:

Mouth – The teeth bite and chew food into a soft substance that is easy to swallow. Chewing mixes the food with watery saliva from six salivary glands around the mouth and face.

Esophagus - The esophagus or (gullet) is a muscular tube. It takes food from the throat and pushes it down through the neck and into the stomach. It moves food by waves of muscle contractions, called peristalsis.

Stomach- The stomach has thick muscles in its wall, which contracts to mash food into a "sloppy soup". The stomach produces strong digestive juices that attack the food in a chemical way, breaking down and dissolving its nutrients.

Pancreas -The pancreas, like the stomach, makes powerful digestive juices called enzymes which help to digest food further as it enters the small intestines.

Gall Bladder - This small bag-like part is tucked under the liver. It stores a fluid called bile, which is made in the liver. As food from a meal arrives in the small intestine, bile flows from the gall bladder along the bile duct into the intestine. It helps to digest fatty foods and also contains wastes for removal.

Small Intestine- This part of the tract is narrow but very long, about 20 feet. In the small intestine, more enzymes continue the chemical attack on food. Finally, the nutrients are small enough to pass through the lining of the small intestine and into the blood. These nutrients are then carried away to the liver and other body parts to be processed, stored and distributed.

Liver -Blood from the intestines flows to the liver, carrying nutrients, vitamins and minerals, and other products from digestion. The liver stores some nutrients, changes them from one form to another, and then releases them into the blood according to the activities and needs of the body.

Large Intestine - Any useful substance in the leftovers, such as spare water and body minerals are absorbed through the walls of the large intestine and back into the blood. The remains are formed into brown, semi-solid feces that is ready to be removed from the body.

Rectum & Anus- The end of the large intestine and the next part of the tract, the rectum, stores the feces. These are finally squeezed through a ring of muscles (the anus) and out of the body.

Carbohydrates

The building block of every carbohydrate is the sugar molecule, composed of carbon, hydrogen and oxygen. Depending on a given carb's complexity, it may have dozens or hundreds of chained molecules. Some carb chains are straight, while others split into intricate branches. Our digestive systems goal is simple; breakdown these sugar chains into singular molecules, which are then small enough to pass into the blood stream. Digestible carbs turn into glucose (blood sugar), providing us with energy. As these sugar molecules enter the blood, our pancreas kicks out the hormone insulin, which signals our cells to absorb those molecules for either immediate energy or storage.

The unused sugars are converted into glycogen, or fatty acids, which can be stored as body fat. As it relates to weight loss or gain, the bodily arithmetic is simple: a carb deficit will force your body to access its energy surplus (fat cells), leading to weight loss, while a carb surplus means those extra sugars get converted to glycogen and stores as fat. A bit of strategy pays off when it comes to carbs. Keep in mind, all carbs are not the same. There are simple carbs, complex carbs and others sources that are almost all fiber. What should be considered are the type, timing and amount, depending on the individual's body type and goals.

Simple Carbs - Simple carbs bite your system fast, load the blood stream up with glycogen, spike your insulin and have an instantaneous effect. They come from sugar sources as well as elements that are rapidly made into sugar sources, such as refined flour (white bread products). There are also artificial "knock offs" such as high fructose corn syrup which are processed just like regular white sugar. Simple carbs do have some nutritional value, but it's generally minimal and should be taken sparingly. A small amount can be helpful in getting your body going in the morning and may consist of a small glass of juice. They also come in handy right after a hard workout, when you want to increase glycogen to the muscles. Outside of these two timeframes, simple carbs should be eaten very sparingly. The excess sugars contribute to the increase in body fat, obesity, diabetes and heart disease, along with reduced functions in immunity, increases in general fatigue, lack of focus and headaches.

Complex Carbs- Complex carbs are the "good" kind, they release their energy over a much longer time span, providing a prolonged burn. They can be eaten on a consistent basis and provide numerous benefits. The starchy carbs found in this category, such as bananas, corn, potatoes and beans are considered a resistant starch in that they're not immediately converted to sugar, and they score low on the glycemic index. These carbs are digested slowly, keeping blood sugar levels stable. The body also uses energy to digest this category of carbs, increasing the body's non-exercise activity thermogenesis response, also known as NEAT. This type of thermogenesis includes any activities the body completes outside of exercise, which burns calories and includes necessary functions such as respiration and digestion.

Fiber Factor -Some carbs are almost all fiber. If you want to stay lean, these sources help cleanse your system and slow down digestion. Fiber in food helps prevent those undesirable spikes in blood sugar levels, helps stabilize the appetite and provides an even, steady flow of energy. The one time you really want to avoid fibers is right after an intense workout. At this point, you don't want to slow digestion and absorption; you want to speed it up instead. Excess fiber can block some nutrients from being absorbed, negating the important effects of repair and recover from important nutrient ingestion after a workout. The bottom line is to increase your fiber intake but avoid ingesting it during the first few hours post-workout.

Carb Cutting - Cutting back on carb intake can be an effective way to drop a few pounds of body weight, but it should be viewed as a short term cyclical tool. The diets that have long term, strict carb reduction of elimination eventually cause large decreases in metabolism, performance and brain function, and cannot be sustained on a permanent basis. Training inevitably begins to suffer, as carbs are a primary subtrate needed for performance and exercise and eventually, vital NEAT functions begin to decline, which can be dangerous for the body's survival.

Type of Carbs	Key Source	Bodily Absorption	Timing
Fast Digesting	Sugar	Fast And Strong	Take Post Workout to Encourage Maximum Muscle Building
Fructose High Fructose Corn Syrup	Fruit Juice Soda	Fairly Fast	Avoid as Fructose Must Be Processed By The Liver And is More Likely To Be Stored as Body Fat
Starchy	Pasta White Bagel Potato White Bread Pancakes White Rice	Fairly Fast	Best Time for These Carbs is Thirty Minutes Post Workout
Vegetables Fruit	Broccoli	Minimal	Low Calories & High Fiber Content Make For Slower Absorption
Lentils & Beans	Lentils Black Bean Kidney Beans	Minimal	Moderate Calories And Very High Fiber Content Make For Slower Absorption
Fiber	Whole Grain Fruits Vegetables Lentils Beans	Minimal	Avoid Post Workout, Emphasize at Other Meals of the Day
Complex	Oatmeal Brown Rice Whole Wheat Bread	Minimal	These Post Workout Carb Should Round Out Your Carb Allotment Consume Them Earlier in the Day

Protein - Protein is a very important macronutrient, it's made up of amino acids, which are the building blocks for tissue repair, muscle growth, and regeneration of all cells of the body. The brain requires protein for development as well. Seafood, eggs and lean meats provide the brain with amino acids that develop neurotransmitters. Well-fed neurotransmitters function at a high efficiency rate and keep the brain sharp. Game meats and organic meats should be your first choice over domestic animals and non-organic meats. Domestic meats have higher levels of adipose fat than game meats, which can slow down blood supply to the brain. As for fish, consume wild caught over farm raised. Free range eggs, chicken, turkey, organic grass fed beef and wild caught fish are some of the best sources of protein, as they contain all the essential amino acids needed to perform all the duties listed prior. It's important to eat as much organic foods as possible because conventionally raised animals and poultry contain a vast array of antibiotics, hormones and pesticides that will wreak havoc on the endocrine system, metabolism and overall health. Avoiding processed meats liked deli slices, is also important since they contain harmful preservatives and unhealthy chemical additives; including hormones, steroids and pesticides.

Many medical experts theorize that these chemicals are the source of numerous medical conditions. If you happen to be a vegetarian, then you can find complete proteins form certain plants like spirubina, soy (fermented only), hemp, and certain grains like buckwheat, quinoa and amaranth. Combining beans, grains and seeds will also form a complete protein. Also, keep in mind that too much protein intake may cause problems should you have an existing liver or kidney disorder. The excess ingested protein that is above the body's daily need must be broken down by the liver to be used for energy (deamination). When deamination occurs, toxins derived from this excess ingested protein may compound any existing liver and/or kidney damage. On high protein diet, excessive urea can be found in urine. This indicates that the protein ingestion is far too high.

Fats – Not all fats are the same. Believe it or not, but fat is a vital component of a healthy diet. You just have to make sure to eat the right kinds of fat. There are two types; saturated and unsaturated fat. Saturated fats, "dumb fats" for example, possess tightly packed molecules that slow blood flow to the brain, raises bad cholesterol levels, and increases the chances of heart disease. They mostly come from red meat, fried foods, cooking oil, cheese, butter, margarine, potato chips, bacon and muffins.

Unsaturated fats, "smart fats", are extremely beneficial to the body and brain health, they actually tend to lower bad cholesterol levels and decrease the chances of heart disease. Those fats come from salmon, tuna, sardines, nuts, soy, flax seed oil, almonds, olives, avocados and seeds. Fat should make up twenty to twenty-five percent of your total calorie intake. Just make sure to consume mostly "smart fats", the unsaturated kind and stay away from fast food places to avoid saturated fats that is in most junk food.

DIETS VS. REGIMEN

Most crash diets out there never tend to work in a long run. So eating like a bird or starving yourself is never a good idea. You might lose a few pounds at first, but very soon your body is going to slow down its' metabolism and will try to hold onto every calorie to preserve energy, simply because it doesn't know when the next meal is coming. So, when you finish your diet and get back to your normal eating habits, your metabolism is still running at a snail's pace, that's why most people get their original weight back very quickly, if not more. The goal here is to achieve the results you want and maintain them for the rest of your life. Like I mentioned earlier, you need to develop a lifetime of healthy eating habits, and commit to a regimen you can be comfortable with. In order to speed up your metabolism and keep it at the highest peak, you should consume about five medium size meals a day that will consist of lean protein, vegetables, fruits, nuts, seeds and dairy every two and a half to three hours. This will let your body know that it will be fed regularly and there's no reason to store fat. Also, try to keep all your meals within the ten hour window, for example: if your first meal of the day is at nine A.M., then your last meal of the day should be at seven P.M. That will give your body a fourteen hour break without any food and plenty of time to burn some fat until the next day.

Every meal should be in a range of five to six hundred calories each. Try to consume one to one and a half grams of protein per pound of your desired body weight. So, if you are a 200 pound man, whose desired body weight is 170 pounds, you should be consuming 170 to 250 grams of protein daily and divide the rest of the calories between complex carbs and unsaturated fats. Once you establish your regimen and you feel like you want to lose weight, take out 300 to 500 calories from your daily intake. If you're trying to build muscle and gain a few pounds, add 300 to 500 calories into your daily intake. But in any case, lean protein should be the main ingredient of your every meal.

If you happen to spin out of control on the weekend, it's no big deal. Logically, there's no reason why your regimen should end with a single slipup. What's the worst that can happen? It sets you back a day or two. What you do six days a week should matter more than what happened on the seventh. In other words, it's okay to give yourself an occasional break in the form of a cheat meal. Just as long as you don't get carried away and get back on the wagon the very next day. So if you must have an occasional cheat meal, I recommend having it the night before your toughest workout. The extra calories, combined with your improved mood, can make that training session more productive.

Power Foods

Whether you're looking to lose weight or add muscle mass, you won't be reaching your goal anytime soon, unless you fuel your body with the right stuff. You're what you eat, and the diet you embrace is as important as training. Therefore, no matter how hard you push yourself during exercise, if you fail to properly address your nutritional needs, the failure is bound to follow. As a result, here are some of the best foods for building muscle mass, performance and total health.

Milk

Milk scores high on the best food list for many reasons. For starters, milk is one of the best post-workout meals because it has water, protein, calcium and natural sugar to help you speed up recovery and the rebuilding process. Furthermore, it's the ideal snacking option, full of casein proteins which help with digestion. Shoot for about two or three cups a day. To bulk up, opt for whole milk. But if weight loss is more important, then have low fat or skim variety.

Eggs

Eggs are a major source of high quality protein, which is what your body needs to build muscle. Eggs are also jam-packed with antioxidants - key for keeping your eyes in top shape. They're also a major source of choline, scientifically proven to boost brain function and health. But there's a catch. Egg yolk scores high in cholesterol; consequently, try to limit your intake to no more than five eggs per week or just simply go for egg whites instead.

Oatmeal

Oatmeal reduces inflammation, tames cholesterol levels and boosts overall heart health, plus provides a sustained source of energy. It's also a good source of fiber at approximately eight grams per serving. Steer clear of some instant oatmeal, as this is often jam-packed with sugars and other artificial ingredients.

Almonds

Almonds are one of the calorie densest foods on the planet with about seventy calories for merely twenty of the nuts. Therefore, most calories conscience dieters avoid them. But that's a big loss. Almonds are a great source of monounsaturated fats, which are essential for optimum heart health. They're also rich in protein and fiber - approximately six grams of protein and three grams of fiber per serving.

Salmon

Salmon is one of the best sources for lean protein - approximately twenty grams for a three ounce serving. And it doesn't stop there; salmon is full of omega-3 fatty acids, great for heart health and decreasing muscle inflammation.

Lentils

When it comes to finding the best low fat source for iron, look no further than these powerful pulses. Iron is key for optimum health. It helps blood deliver the maximum amount of oxygen to your body and working muscles so that your cells can generate more energy. Make sure to consume lentils with a good source of vitamin C, such as a glass of fresh juice, raw tomatoes, or peppers to facilitate iron absorption.

Avocados

Avocados are also a superb source of healthy fats (monounstaturated and omega-3s) which are essential for lowering cholesterol levels and reducing the risk of heart disease. They're also packed with a variety of vitamins - about twenty to be exact. One half of an avocado has approximately 160 calories and 14 grams of fat and 7 grams of fiber.

Acai Berry

Acai is a Brazilian berry that is low in sugar and tastes like a mixture of red wine and chocolate. Although the acai berry resembles a large blueberry, only the outermost layer of acai berries are edible. It's believed to contain up to twenty times the amount of antioxidants found in grapes, pomegranates, and blueberries. Acai berries are rich in the omega fats aleic and linoleic acids, which can boost heart health and help with hair loss.

Star Fruit

Each star fruit has just thirty calories and is loaded with antioxidants and flavonoids. It's high in vitamin A, which is a vitamin that's crucial to cellular health because it makes cells resistant to free radicals. It's also high in iron and great source of vitamin C. Star fruit is also loaded with fiber, which speeds transit time, aides digestion and helps control body weight.

Guava

Guava is often referred to as a "super-fruit", it's packed with high levels of antioxidants and vitamins. Guava is one of the best sources of vitamin C. It has five times more vitamin C than an orange. Plus guava seeds are rich in omego-3 and omega- 6 fatty acids. It's also loaded with heart-healthy benefits and has been proven to keep blood pressure in check and reduce the risk of cancer.

Rambutan

Rambutan is extremely low in calories, with just seven calories per fruit. It's loaded with vitamins A and C, magnesium, potassium, zinc, and fiber. Rambutan also helps lowering blood pressure and is a natural curative against gastrointestinal distress as well.

Hydration

Don't underestimate the role that water plays in your body. Drinking eight glasses of water daily should be just as important as breathing. It's the most vital nutrient than all of the rest. Therefore, maintaining hydration is a very important part of healthy living. For example: You can survive for forty days without food, but not more than a week without water. Your body consists of about sixty percent water. If the water in your body is reduced by twenty percent, you're dead. Proper water intake helps to eliminate waste products from the body. It delivers nutrients to muscles, regulates the pattern of your heart rate, it helps manage blood pressure and alleviates hunger pains.

The mechanism for thirst are so weak, that we confuse it for hunger. By drinking more water, you can noticeably decrease your calorie intake.

In other words, water helps you burn more calories and eat less. As far as energy goes, dehydration will definitely have a negative effect on your performance. For every one percent body mass you can lose through sweat, your heart rate ticks up three beats a minute, which means it has to work harder. If you stay hydrated, it helps your body hold in more water, so your heart has to work less to pump the blood to muscles. Keeping your heart rate low allows you to exercise with a higher intensity. The key is to hydrate before your workout, not just during. As for how much to drink, use your next workout to figure it out:

Weigh yourself before and after the exercise, and note how much "sweat weight" you lost. Then before your next workout, be sure to take in that weight in liquid. So, if you haven't been drinking enough water, start now and try to carry a water bottle with you whenever you can.

Meal Strategies

Now that you know how to eat right, it's time to start creating your own meals. Just concentrate on two things and you'll be alright. Read the nutrition labels on food packages and pay close attention to the calories per serving. By now, you are well aware of what to put in your body and what to banish completely. With some practice down the line, you won't even have to think about what to eat, it will just come natural. Here are some examples for your weekly meal schedule.

	Monday
Breakfast:	Steel-cut oatmeal with low fat milk and a handfull of fresh raspberries
Lunch:	Tuna on a whole-wheat wrap with pickles, onions, tomatoes, fat free mayo and a hand full of pistachios
Snack:	Granola bar with a cup of acai berries
Dinner:	Chicken breast with broccoli, baked potato, and a spoon of extra-virgin olive oil
	Tuesday
Breakfast:	Greek yogurt with fresh blueberries, almonds and a peach
Lunch:	Grilled turkey sandwich on a whole-wheat bread with lettuce, tomatoes, pickles, onions, mustard and a piece of fresh papaya
Snack:	Hummus with whole wheat crackers and sliced cucumbers
Dinner:	Red snapper with quinoa, green beans and asparagus

	Wednesday
Breakfast:	Organic peanut butter on whole wheat bread and a banana
Lunch:	Tuscan salad with grilled salmon, sun dried tomatoes, arugula, asparagus, low fat mozzarella cheese, roasted peppers, reduced fat balsamic dressing and 1/2 cup of dried dates
Snack:	Low fat cheddar cheese cubes with 1/2 cup of walnuts
Dinner:	Grass fed beef tenderloin with cooked cabbage, onions, red and green peppers, mushrooms and tomato sauce
	Thursday
Breakfast:	Boiled eggs with whole wheat crackers, low fat mayo and an apple
Lunch:	Greek salad with grilled chicken breast, red and green bell peppers, cucumber, celery, olives, low fat dressing, 2 tablespoons of reduced fat feta cheese and 1/2 a cup of dried apricots
Snack:	Boiled corn on the cobb with fat free butter and a hand full of Brazil nuts
Dinner:	Tilapia with brown rice, cauliflower, wedge lemon, and a spoon of extra virgin olive oil

	Friday
Breakfast:	Cottage cheese with fresh strawberries and a 1/4 of a cantaloupe
Lunch:	Thai shrimp salad with cabbage, red cabbage, onions, bean sprouts, ginger salad dressing, a hand full of almonds and a glass of pomegranate juice
Snack:	Sticks of fresh celery with a spoon of organic peanut-butter and 1/2 a cup of dried raisins
Dinner:	Top round steak with sweet potato, raw spinach salad and a spoon of balsamic vinegar
	Saturday
Breakfast:	Vegetable omelet on a whole wheat wrap and a glass of freshly squeezed orange juice
Lunch:	Half an avocado stuffed with lobster, green bell peppers, red onions, cucumbers, fresh orange segments, lemon juice, low fat Greek yogurt and 1/4 of watermelon
Snack:	Baked eggplant slices with low fat mozzarella cheese and cherry tomatoes
Dinner:	Turkey breast with barley, mushrooms, red peppers and onions

	Sunday
Breakfast:	Fresh fruit salad of your choice with granola and dried raisins
Lunch:	Buffalo burger on a whole wheat bun with pickles, onions, tomatoes, mushrooms, ketchup or mustard and cup of fresh cherries
Snack:	Fresh baby carrots with walnuts and a spoonful of organic honey
Dinner:	Shrimp and scallops with whole wheat pasta, zucchini, yellow squash, low fat Parmesan cheese and a spoon of extra virgin olive oil

Those are just some examples you can use, but feel free to create your own meals by using your imagination. So have fun on your journey, and remember, all your goals are within your reach!

Seva

About The Author

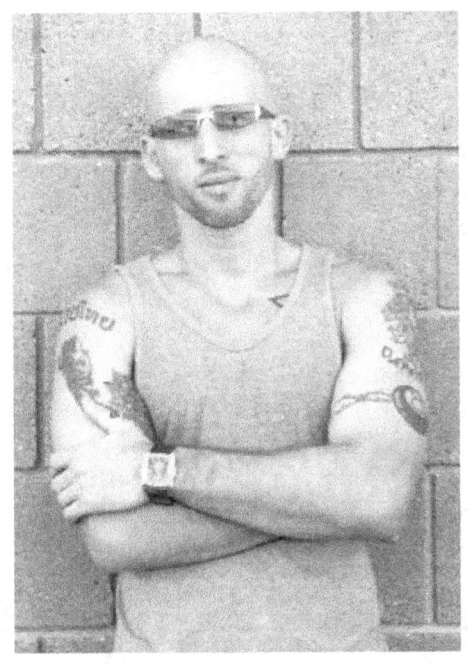

Vsevolod Berkolayko is a professional kickboxer and a winner of a K-1 World Championship Tournament. He is a co-author of "Betrayed Soul" and "Commrades" film scripts, which he wrote inside prison walls along with the following manuscript. He is planning to get back into the 'fighting game' upon his release in 2015.

We Help You Self-Publish Your Book

Crystell Publications can help you self-publish your novel. Regardless of your status, our team will help you get to print. Our BLOW OUT prices are for serious authors only. **Don't have all your money? ....** **No Problem!** *Ask About our Payment Plans*

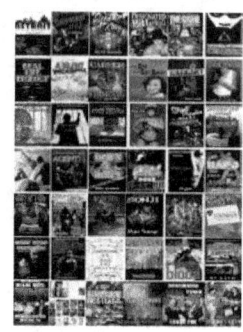

Crystal Perkins-Stell, MHR
Essence Magazine Bestseller
We Give You Books!
PO BOX 8044 / Edmond – OK 73083
www.crystalstell.com
(405) 414-3991

Our competitor's Cheapest Plans-
AuthorHouse Legacy Plan $1299.00- 8 books **Xilibris** Professional Plan $1249.00
iUniverse Premier Plan $1299.00-5 bks   10 bks

Hey! Stop Wishing, and get your book to print NOW!!!

–Recession Big Flex Options 100 Books–					
Option A	**Option B**	**Option C**	**Option D**	**E-Book**	**Option F**
$1399.00	**$1299.00**	**$1199.00**	**$839.00**	**$695.00**	**$775.00**
255-275	205-250	200 -80	75 - 60	255 pages	50 or less

Grind Plans 25 & E-Book	**Hustle Hard**	**Respect The Code**	**313 Deal**
Order Extra Books	**$899.00**	**$869.00**	**$839.00**
	255-275pg	250 -205	200 -80

Insanity Plans 2 Books & E-Book & POD	**Psycho**	**Spastic**	**Mental**
Extra Books Can Be Ordered	**$759.00**	**$659.00**	**$559.00**
	225-250pg	200-220	199- 100

All Manuscript Options except the E-Books include:
2 Proofs–Publisher & Printer, Mink Magazine Subscription, Free Advertisement, Book Cover, ISBN #, Conversion, Typeset, Correspondence, Masters, 8 hrs Consultation

$100.00 E-book upload only   **$75** Can't afford edits, Spell-check
$275.00-Book covers/Authors input   **$499** Flat Rate Edits Exceeds 210 add 1.50
$269.00-Book covers/ templates   **$200**-Typeset Book Format PDF File
$190.00 and up Websites   **$200 and up** / Type Manuscript Call for details
$375.00, book trailers on Youtube

We're Killing The Game.
No more paying Vanity Presses $8 to $10 per book! We Give You Books @ Cost. **We Offer Editing For An Extra Fee- If Waved, We Print What You Submit!** These titles are done by self-published authors. They are not published by nor signed to Crystell Publications.